T0257783

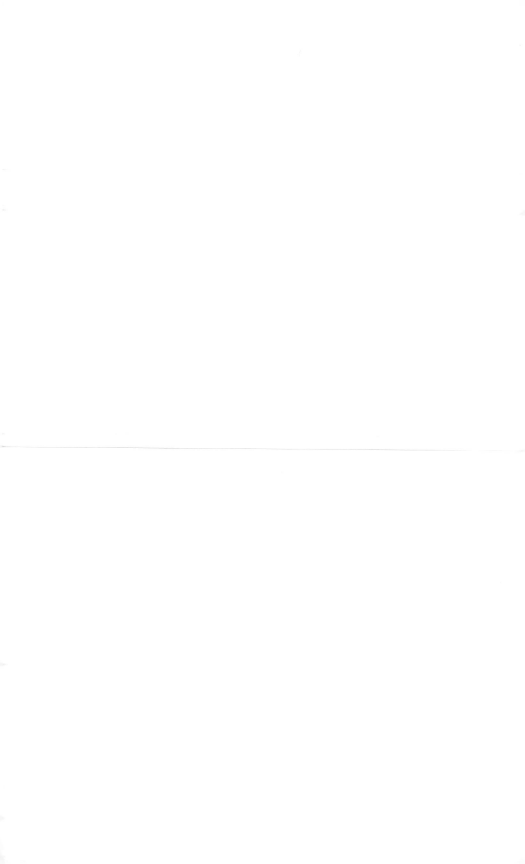

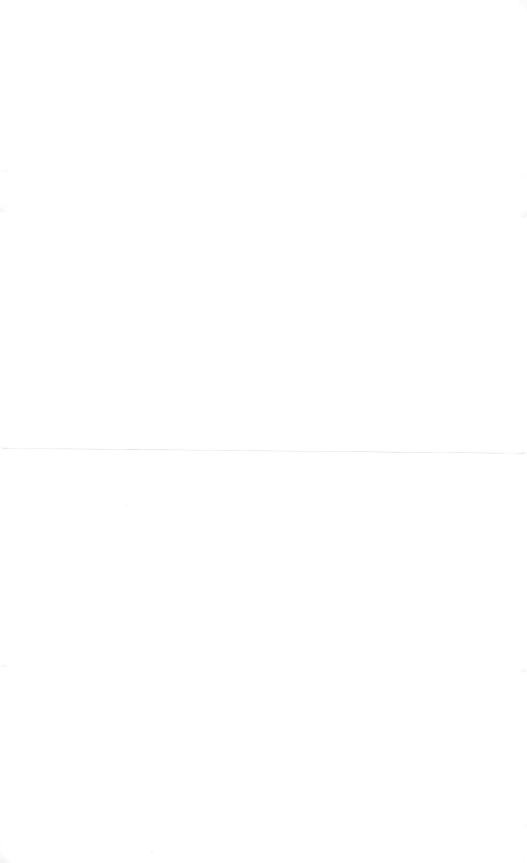

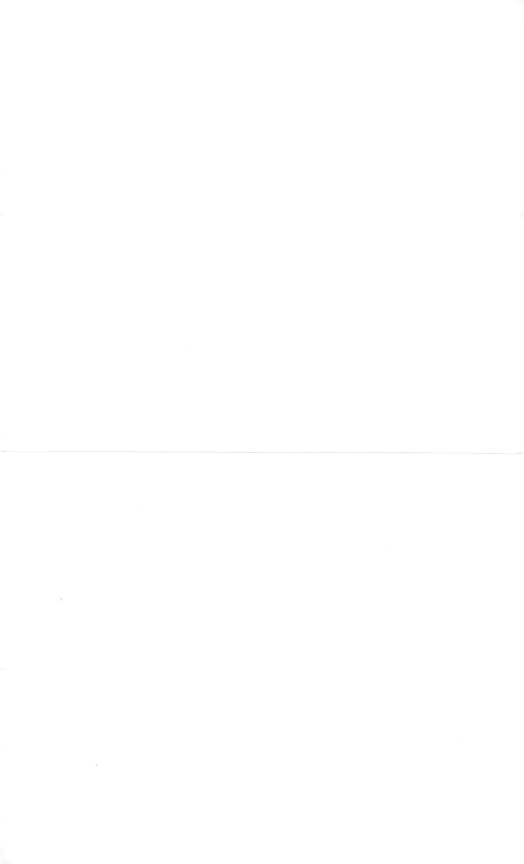

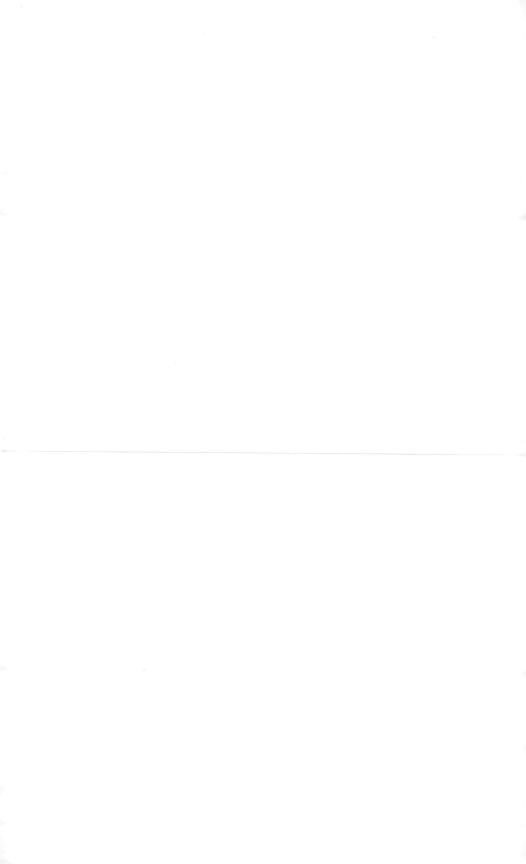

Handbook of Regenerative Medicine and Tissue Engineering

Volume II

Handbook of Regenerative Medicine and Tissue Engineering
Volume II

Edited by **Shay Fisher**

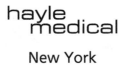

New York

Published by Hayle Medical,
30 West, 37th Street, Suite 612,
New York, NY 10018, USA
www.haylemedical.com

Handbook of Regenerative Medicine and Tissue Engineering
Volume II
Edited by Shay Fisher

© 2015 Hayle Medical

International Standard Book Number: 978-1-63241-244-7 (Hardback)

This book contains information obtained from authentic and highly regarded sources. Copyright for all individual chapters remain with the respective authors as indicated. A wide variety of references are listed. Permission and sources are indicated; for detailed attributions, please refer to the permissions page. Reasonable efforts have been made to publish reliable data and information, but the authors, editors and publisher cannot assume any responsibility for the validity of all materials or the consequences of their use.

The publisher's policy is to use permanent paper from mills that operate a sustainable forestry policy. Furthermore, the publisher ensures that the text paper and cover boards used have met acceptable environmental accreditation standards.

Trademark Notice: Registered trademark of products or corporate names are used only for explanation and identification without intent to infringe.

Printed in the United States of America.

Contents

Permissions

List of Contributors

Preface

Over the recent decade, advancements and applications have progressed exponentially. This has led to the increased interest in this field and projects are being conducted to enhance knowledge. The main objective of this book is to present some of the critical challenges and provide insights into possible solutions. This book will answer the varied questions that arise in the field and also provide an increased scope for furthering studies.

The basic concept of regenerative medicine and tissue engineering is intriguing for physicians and scientists as it involves healing tissues or organ defects that the present medical practice finds difficult or impossible to cure. Tissue engineering involves cells, materials methods and engineering supported by appropriate physiochemical and biological factors to enhance or replace biologic functions. Regenerative medicine is a new division of medicine which aims to change the course of chronic disease and regenerate failing organ systems lost due to damage, age, disease and congenital defects. This book reflects state-of-the-art of these two disciplines at this time, as well as their therapeutic application. It discusses various topics under scaffolds and matrices. This book provides as a reference for physicians, scientists and students and as an explanatory analysis for individuals in pharmaceuticals and biotech companies.

I hope that this book, with its visionary approach, will be a valuable addition and will promote interest among readers. Each of the authors has provided their extraordinary competence in their specific fields by providing different perspectives as they come from diverse nations and regions. I thank them for their contributions.

Editor

Scaffolds and Matrices

Biomaterials for Cardiac Tissue Engineering

M. Arnal-Pastor, J. C. Chachques,
M. Monleón Pradas and A. Vallés-Lluch

Additional information is available at the end of the chapter

1. Introduction

1.1. Cardiovascular diseases

Cardiovascular diseases (CVD) are a leading death cause in developed countries (1 of every 3 deaths in the United States in 2008) [1]. Changes in diet and habits are causing CVD to become major mortality pathologies in developing countries too [2] (they are already responsible for a 30% of the world deaths). This group of diseases constitutes a great burden for the national health systems, consuming great percentages of the health systems budgets. In the particular case of the coronary heart diseases (CHD), 3,8 million men and 3,4 million women die a year worldwide because of them [3]. In the United States 1 of every 6 deaths in 2008 was caused by CHD [1].

The heart is a complex organ that pumps 7000 liters of blood to all the tissues in the body per day [4]. This pumping function precisely determines its anatomy. Heart tissue basically is formed by cardiac myocytes (contractile elements) [5], smooth muscle cells, fibroblasts, blood vessels, nerves and the extracellular matrix components (cardiac interstitium and collagen) [6] organized in a very particular way. Myocytes form muscular fibers with changing orientation across the ventricular wall up to 180° [7]. At the same time, muscular fibers are organized into myocardial laminas 4-6 myocytes thick separated from neighboring laminas by extracellular collagen [8]. The particular arrangement of the ventricular myocytes influence the mechanical and electrical function of the heart and small changes in it can lead to severe changes in these functions [9].

The extracellular matrix (ECM) connects the cells into a 3D architecture allowing the coupling of the forces produced by the myocytes. The anatomical model proposed by Torrent-Guasp [8], which considers the heart one muscle band plied in a double helical loop, explains how the ventricles contract and get an efficient pumping in every heart beat, achieving an ejection fraction of the 60% when sarcomeres individually contract 15% only [10].

Myocytes are intimately connected, forming a functional syncytium [8]. Each myocardial cell is coupled in average to 9,1 ± 2,2 [11] myocytes, by 99 [12] gap junctions where the transfer of ionic currents takes place. Gap junctions are a specialized form of cell connection; they are formed by a cluster of ionic channels essential to the rapid propagation of the action potential. The action potential is the electrical impulse responsible for the contraction of the cells [13]. A proper electrical coupling of the cells is critical to avoid arrhythmias and reentries and essential for the contraction to spread as a wave front.

Acute myocardial infarction (AMI) occurs when a coronary artery is clogged, in 80% of the cases, by coronary atherosclerosis with superimposed luminal thrombus [14]. This occlusion leaves the downstream zone of the heart without blood supply, what means lack of oxygen, nutrients and metabolites wash for the affected zone. As a consequence, the aerobic metabolism changes to anaerobic glycolysis [14], leading to a decrease in the pH and reduction in the contractile function. Within 20 to 40 minutes without blood supply cells start to die and as times passes more myocardial tissue is compromised. There is also a zone of the heart affected by the infarction, where myocytes remain viable but lower their activity to reduce the metabolism and oxygen consumption to survive under hypoxic conditions; they can recover their contractibility after revascularization [15].

Clinical practices aim to limit the severity and extension of the AMI by rapidly restoring the blood flow (reperfusion), alleviating the oxygen demand [16] and reducing reperfusion injury. This can be done with different treatments or combinations of them. Pharmacological approaches involve the use of anticoagulant therapies and thrombolytic drugs to eliminate the clot. Vasodilatators like nitrates are also used to favor the dilation of the vessels, aspirin to avoid platelet aggregation, betabloqueants to reduce the heart pace, as well as morphine to reduce the pain are employed. Another group of therapies are the percutaneous coronary interventions; they physically reopen the vessel via catheterization. There are different techniques: the regular angioplasty uses a catheter with a balloon that is inflated in the place of the thrombus to reopen the lumen [17], or allows the permanent implantation of a stent in the vessel to keep it open. There is a wide variety of these devices depending on their composition, whether they release drugs or are biodegradable or not, etc [18, 19].

These therapies restore the blood flow to the infarcted zone; but reperfusion therapy is not exempt of risks: it is a complex process that can induce apoptosis by the microenvironmental changes that the recovery of the blood supply induces (formation of free radicals, calcium release, neutrophils, etc.) [20]. So it has to be done carefully and there is always a compromise between limiting the infarction extension due to the time without oxygen and the induced apoptosis due to the reperfusion. Reperfusion done soon after the onset of the ischemia is very advantageous, saving more tissue by restoring the blood flow than the tissue that will be lost because of the toxic substances released in the reperfusion. All the aforementioned treatments basically limit the damage of the acute episode but do not regenerate the damaged tissue and do not avoid the subsequent ventricular remodeling following an AMI.

In the infarcted area there is a great number of dead myocytes, and the host response to the injury consists in activating the inflammatory response and producing cytokines [21]. Thereupon neutrophils, monocytes and macrophages migrate into this area to remove the necrotic tissue [22]. Then, matrix metalloproteases (MMPs) are activated, which have a deleterious effect on the collagen matrix of the heart and in the surrounding coronary vasculature by degrading them [23]. The weakening of the collagen leads to wall thinning and ventricular dilation, as well as mural realignment of myocytes bundles [24]. After the inflammatory phase and the resorption of the necrotic tissue, there is an increase in the deposition of cross-linked collagen in the infarcted area that leads to scar tissue formation. During the remodelling process a change in the collagen composition occurs, the type I collagen fraction is reduced from 80% to 40% and the collagen III is increased [25].

Against what it was thought, this scar is a living tissue with a fibroblast-like cell population nourished by a neovasculature; these cells regulate the collagen turnover of the scar tissue [22]. The scar tissue has a reduced or absent contractility as compared with the original healthy myocardium [26], what leads to a reduction in the overall cardiac function [27].

The remodeling process initially is a compensatory mechanism to overcome the loss of contractile tissue. But with time this adaptative process of overload becomes maladaptative [15]. To compensate the additional effort, the remaining beating tissue hypertrophies trying to overcome the reduction in the cardiac function. This overload leads to myocyte slippage and fibrotic interstitial growth and to a degenerating process that may end in heart failure. The heart remodeling produces in the ventricles a set of anatomical and functional changes, including increased wall stress, slimming of the wall, chamber dilation, increase of the sphericity, and a significant loss of cardiac function.

The ventricular shape change from elliptical to spherical reduces its ejection fraction, because of a change in the apical loop fiber orientation [28]. Another problem caused by the shape change is that the papillary muscles are separated, what leads to regurgitation, contributing to the overload of the heart [24]. Besides, remodeled hearts are more prone to suffer arrhythmias as the membrane potential is altered and because of the interstitial fibrotic growth that may affect conductivity [15].

The end stage of the degeneration is the heart failure, when the heart is unable to pump enough blood to match the metabolic needs of the tissues. Current treatments aim to avoid reaching this point. Pharmacological treatments aspire to reduce the work load and to protect the cardiac tissues from the accumulated harmful substances [29]. Surgical therapy involves different techniques with different objectives: to restore a proper blood flow in areas that lack it (bypass surgery), to restore the normal elliptical geometry (Dor and Batista procedures), to restore the wall stress to normal (Dynamic Cardiomyoplasty), to limit the pathologic dilation, etc [10].

1.2. Cell therapy and cardiac tissue engineering

For many years, the heart has been considered a fully differentiated organ, with no myocyte regeneration after birth [30]. Recently it has been proved that myocytes have a limited regenerative capacity, around 1% of the cells per year at the age of 20 and it is reduced to 0,3%

at the age of 75 [31]. This regenerative capacity is achieved thanks to a small population of cardiac stem cells [32]. Nevertheless, their regenerative capacity is limited and in any case it is not enough to regenerate the heart if it suffers severe damage, like the one provoked by a myocardial infarction. New therapies under development like cell therapy or tissue engineering, aim to boost this limited regenerative potential of the native tissue by employing cells, drugs, factors or patches.

The aim of cardiac cell therapy is to heal the damaged infarcted tissue by the implantation of cells into or onto the pathologic myocardium by different techniques (figure 1 a). In tissue engineering strategies, different types of cells have been combined with materials and with bioactive molecules if necessary to again try to recover the injured tissue. The employed materials will support cells, provide them 3D organization, protect them, stimulate and guide its growth, maintain them in the site of interest, etc.; in sum, they will act as an artificial extracellular matrix during the regeneration process. But the use of materials either injectable, or *ex vivo* conformed (gels –patches- or scaffolds) (figure 1 b) has an additional and important effect: the implantation of a material in the scarred ventricular wall, increases its thickness and by Laplace's law, this increase leads to a reduction in the wall stress. This side-effect could be by itself very positive, even although regeneration did not arrive to happen, to limit ventricular remodeling and improve the quality of life of cardiac patients [29].

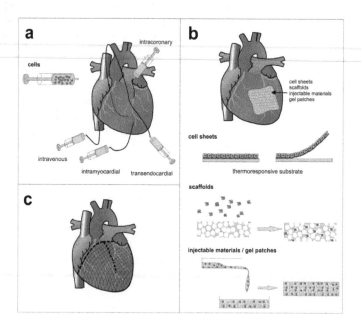

Figure 1. (a) Classical cell therapy in the heart (*freely inspired* in Strauer BE, Kornowski R, *Circulation* 2003; 107: 929-934). (b) Tissue engineering approaches with cell sheets, scaffolds or injectable materials (*freely inspired in* Masuda S *et al*, *Adv. Drug Del. Revs* 2008; 60(2): 277-85). (c) Ventricular restrain device.

2. Cardiomyoplasty

2.1. Need for cell cardiomyoplasty

Cardiomyoplasty has evolved from "dynamic" to "cellular cardiomyoplasty". The term dynamic cardiomyoplasty is referred to a surgical procedure developed in 1987 [33] to wrap the heart with the latissimus dorsi muscle, aiming to support the heart beating and limit the remodeling. Nevertheless, the obtained results were not as good as expected. With the advances in cell therapy, cellular cardiomyoplasty appeared as a promising therapeutical approach. This name encloses the therapies that use the injection of cells, from different origins, directly into the heart to try to obtain an improvement in the reduced heart function after an ischemic insult (figure 1 a).

The injected cells are envisaged to induce angiogenesis, inhibit apoptosis, help to recover hibernating myocardium, activate endogenous repair mechanisms, and create new contractile tissue that will replace the damaged one. Also they are expected to reverse the remodeling process that provoked ventricular dilation [34]. Many cells have been employed and the initial promising results obtained in animal models made this technique moved very fast to clinical trials, even if the mechanisms involved in the observed improvements were unknown. Unfortunately, the results obtained from the clinical trials were not as good as expected, and some were contradictory between them. One possible contributing cause to this discrepancy is that studies are carried out in young healthy animals, while patients susceptible to receive these treatments normally are aged people and in many cases with other co-morbidities [35].

Different ways to deliver cells into the damaged heart have been explored: intracoronary infusion (with the hope that cells will migrate through the vessels and be hosted in the infarcted area) or directly into the infarcted area either by intramyocardial or endocardial injection [36], as shown in figure 1 a. The advantage of injecting them directly into the infarcted area is that this will ensure that the cells are delivered in the site of interest.

2.2. Related problematic

Many different cell types have been employed in the numerous studies that have been done. Autologous cell sources are interesting because they do not require immunosuppression treatment of the patient and there is no risk of illness transmission. On the contrary, allogenic cells could be ready to use whenever a patient needs them, but would require immunosuppressive therapy after their implantation, and there is always a remaining risk of illness transmission. Another disadvantage is that prior to implantation cells need to be extracted and expanded. This whole process in some cases may take several weeks, limiting its application in the acute state. Besides, autologous cells coming from patients that suffer other conditions like diabetes or are simply aged, may have limited proliferation and attachment [37].

An important aspect of this technique is the low engraftment into the heart tissue of the supplied cells. The retention of the cells in the heart seems to be determined by the cell type and delivery route [38]. It has been estimated that in humans 50-75 min after intracoronary injection of bone marrow cells only 1,3-2,6% of the injected cells remain in the myocardium

[39]; after 2 hours less than 10% of the injected cells survive [32]. Many causes can be advanced: the heart beats, so cells can easily be pumped out of the heart; the solution in which cells are injected has a low viscosity, so cells can be washed away; the mechanical loss of the cells through the injection hole left by the needle, etc [40]. A different contributing cause to the low cell engraftment is that the injured heart is not a cell-friendly environment, type I collagen fibers have been substituted by type III, which has worse properties in terms of adhesion and promoting angiogenesis, what can induce anoikis [4]. Another problem is cell survival itself. The conditions in the infarcted myocardium are very hostile for the cells: hypoxic conditions (studies show that the survival of injected cells decreases towards the center of the scar), cytokines, inflammatory factors, etc., are present in the damaged myocardium, and can negatively affect the survival of the injected cells. Immunological rejection can be another cause reducing cell survival [41].

An interesting approach is to train cells prior to their implantation for them to resist the hostile conditions they will find in the implantation site. For instance, the resistance to hypoxic conditions is key and needs to be improved even for skeletal myoblasts (which are the cells that have better resistance to lack of oxygen). Privation of glutamine reduces the oxygen consumption rate, what has been proved to improve survival of myoblasts when implanted [42].

The fact that most of the cells did not graft into the host myocardium in the studies performed to date, that there is a very limited transdifferentiation of implanted cells into beating cardiomyocytes (the differentiation reported in animals may have been fusion events between native cardiomyocytes and injected cells [41]), and that a wide range of non-myogenic cells also induce an improvement of the ventricular function [36], suggests that the mechanism leading to this enhancement cannot be only myogenesis regenerating the myocardium. The pathways through which cell implantation induces improvements in cardiac function remain to be elucidated, but different events that can take place simultaneously have been proposed. The most remarkable are the induction of angiogenesis (formation of new vessels) and the improvement in the myocardial perfusion, the reduction of the wall stress because of the increase in cell mass [43] and the paracrine effect of the injected cells [32].

2.3. Cell types investigated

As previously said, many cell types from different origins have been employed: embryonic stem cells, mesenchymal stem cells, bone marrow cells, induced pluripotent stem cells, cardiac stem cells, skeletal myoblasts, umbilical cord blood cells and amniotic fluid stem cells, among others. In what follows the use of these cell types is discussed, with the advantages and disadvantages that each one presents for its application in heart regeneration.

Embryonic Stem Cells (ESC)

ESC can be obtained from the inner mass of an embryo in the blastocyst stage. These cells have the capacity of growing undifferentiated indefinitely, and when they differentiate they can form any cell from the three germ layers. But the use of ESC raises ethical issues, requires immunosuppression, and has the risk to form theratomes. Their use in clinical trials has been limited because of these ethical considerations and risks [36, 44].

A protocol for ESC differentiation into cardiomyocytes and improving their survival when implanted has been established; when these differentiated cells were implanted in rodent models the heart function was improved [45]. In another study in mice, ESC-derived cardiomyocytes implantation reduced the reactive collagen deposition in the ventricular septum, which is one of the remodeling process hallmarks. Nevertheless, the implanted cells were isolated from the host myocardium by scar tissue, although the implanted cardiomyocytes were able to couple functionally to each other [46].

Induced Pluripotent Stem cells (IPS)

Induced pluripotent stem cells are fibroblasts treated with viral factors to recover their pluripotency. Therefore, IPS do not raise the ethical concerns of the ESC. IPS are very interesting because they can be autologous pluripotent cells. However, their application in clinical trials has been limited precisely for the use of viral vectors that may promote malignancy and act as oncogenes [43], as well as for the intrinsic risk of theratomes inherent to their pluripotency [44].

Adult stem cells

These cells have the advantage of being autologous and can be obtained from different sources like bone marrow or adipose tissue. In addition, they can be expanded *in vitro* and do not raise ethical or immunologic problems [47, 48].

Bone marrow cells (BMC) are easily accessible, can be obtained rapidly and have been reported to have certain plasticity. This property allows them to differentiate *in vivo* into cardiomyocytes [26] (although this fact remains controversial [42]). They can also differentiate into cardiomyocytes *in vitro* by supplementing the medium [49]. Studies in animal models demonstrate that the injection of these cells increases neovasculature improving heart function [42]. But the use of BMC is not exempt of risks: intracoronary administration of them can cause microinfarctions due to their big size and irregular shape, making necessary the use of an alternative way of delivery [50]. In clinical trials, results indicated only temporary benefits or no improvement after cell administration [38, 51]. A strategy to enhance the therapeutic efficacy of BMC is to precondition them: BMC treated with growth factors improve the therapeutic effect when implanted and show greater survival rate [52].

Adipose derived stem cells (ASC) can be obtained in great quantity without culturing them. These cells have been implanted in small animal models of AMI and left ventricular function was improved [48]. The underlying mechanisms are unclear, although the hypothesis of a paracrine effect is considered [53]. Clinical trials are ongoing for the implantation of ASCs: PRECISE and APOLLO [54]. These cells are also are under study at the moment in the RECATABI project [55] as part of a strategy that combines them within a three-dimensional polymer scaffold with a peptide gel filling, to lengthen their positive effect and serve as a mechanical support for the dilated ventricle.

Cardiac Stem Cells (CSC)

CSC are undifferentiated cells found in the heart that can become endothelial cells, smooth muscle cells, and functional cardiomyocytes [36]. In undamaged hearts, these cells seem to contribute to the normal self-renewal of the tissue. CSC can be isolated from biopsies and can be expanded *in vitro* [56], although there is a lack of availability from human origin as they are obtained from biopsies. Human CSC injected in mice hearts after infarction led to functional improvement and to support myocardial regeneration [57]. Currently, autologous cardio-sphere-derived cells are being evaluated in the CADUCEUS clinical trial [58].

Skeletal Myoblasts (SM)

SM are cells present in the basal membrane, where they remain in a quiescent state while there is no damage. These cells have better resistance to hypoxic conditions than many other cell types, and can be from autologous origin, but 2 to 3 weeks are necessary to establish and expand myoblasts from skeletal muscle biopsies [36]. These cells are capable to contract; that is the reason why they were expected to attach to the beating cardiomyocytes and contribute to the effective beating by integrating in the working syncytium muscle. Nevertheless, there is no electro-mechanical coupling between the implanted cells and the native cardiomyocytes. This absence of coupling turns the implanted cells into a pro-arrhythmic substrate [44]. The cause for this uncoupling is the lack of the gap junctional protein connexin 43. Therefore, the implantation of a pacemaker or a defibrillator to avoid malignant arrhythmias and sudden death would be necessary when implanting these cells, to obtain a synchronous beating of the heart and the grafted cells [26, 59]. Despite the lack of electro-mechanical coupling of the myoblasts with the host cardiac cells, improvements in the ventricular performance have been observed in animal models, even with a reduced number of grafted cells, suggesting a cytokine-mediated effect [46].

The encouraging preliminary results and its autologous origin made this cell type the first to reach clinical trials. Initial clinical trials carried out with these cells showed symptomatic improvements in the patients, but some of them experienced arrhythmias, making necessary the use of implantable defibrillators [36]. For instance, in the phase II randomized placebo controlled trial MAGIC [60], skeletal myoblasts and a cardioverter defibrillator were implanted during a coronary artery by-pass graft surgery.

Umbilical Cord Blood Cells (UCBC)

UCBC can be easily obtained from the umbilical cord and do not present ethical concerns [42]. These cells have certain plasticity and reduced risk of rejection because they show low immunogenicity [25]. Their injection in animal models has been found to improve their left ventricular function [61].

Amniotic Fluid Stem Cells (AFSC)

Amniotic fluid is extracted for prenatal diagnosis and AFSC are isolated from it. They have many characteristics of ESC and seem to be in an intermediate stage between embryonic and adult stem cells in terms of versatility. Interestingly, these cells do not present ethical concerns and do not present risk of tumorogenicity [62].

Human AFSC have been successfully differentiated into endothelial or cardiac lineages *in vitro*. When these cells were implanted in an immunosupressed rat model, they contributed to attenuate its left ventricular remodeling, to preserve the thickness of the ventricle and to improve cardiac function [63].

3. Cell sheets

The use of cell sheets is based on the fact that when cells are cultured in normal flasks and enzymatically digested to detach them, the adhesive proteins and membrane receptors are disrupted leaving the cell damaged [64]. The alternative is to grow cell sheets and then detach them from the culture surface in a way that keeps the electromechanical connections between the cells and benefits from the fact that cells are kept together by their own deposited ECM, as figure 1 b displays. In that way, cells maintain the adhesion and membrane proteins, as well as the natural pro-survival and maturation environmental cues that the ECM provides [65]. Altogether, this is expected to help them to survive when implanted onto the infarcted myocardium.

Cells can be cultured, for instance, on temperature-responsive poly(N-isopropylacrylamide) (PnIPAAm)-coated plates. PnIPAAm is a hydrophobic polymer at 37ºC, and cells can attach to its surface. When the temperature is lowered, PnIPAAm suffers a transition to a hydrophilic state and this change causes the attachments of the cell monolayer to the surface to disrupt, and the entire cells sheet detaches from the surface [65]. Other materials, such as a thermo-responsive methylcellulose hydrogel, have been used to successfully obtain cell sheets fragments of human amniotic fluid stem cells (hAFSCs) [66]. Results obtained with these cell sheet fragments were superior to those with dissociated cells in terms of heart function, cell retention, proliferation and vascular density. Moreover, cardiomyocyte sheets were found to functionally integrate with the host tissue in a rat myocardial infarct model [67]. New techniques based on patterning with a gelatin stamp the thermo-responsive substrates allow obtaining complex tissue structures with cells having a determined orientation [68].

The muscle mass loss following an infarction is significant, up to 50 g [69], so the amount of cells needed to overcome this loss is obviously not covered with a single sheet of cells. On the other hand, when several layers of cell sheets are superimposed, they are easier to handle. Some groups have tried to obtain thicker grafts by overlapping several monolayer cardiomyocyte sheets, which adhere one to another forming gap junctions and intercellular adhesions within minutes [70]. But this approach poses a problem: as cell sheets lack of vascularization, the maximum thickness that can be achieved by overlapping them is limited to the depth at which diffusion of oxygen and nutrients can take place (a maximum of three cardiomyocyte sheets can be piled up). To try to overcome this problem, three-layer thick cardiomyocyte sheets were implanted in rats at 1-, 2- and 3-day intervals [71]; in the time between transplantations it was assumed that there is enough time for the cell sheet to be vascularized. With this approach constructs of 1 mm were obtained successfully. But anyway, this option is very invasive, so its application in patients might be limited.

A different approach based on the same idea of providing cell-cell connections and ECM to the implanted cells to improve their retention and survival is to implant them as spherical cell-bodies. Human amniotic fluid stem cells (hAFSC) cultured in a methylcellulose hydrogel to form cell aggregates were implanted in immunosuppressed rats as cell-bodies, and cell retention and engraftment were enhanced as compared with disaggregated cells. This enhancement led to functional improvement and limited the progression of heart failure [72].

4. Injectable gels

4.1. Rationale

As previously stated, cell cardiomyoplasty presents problems in terms of cell attachment and survival. Cells usually reside in a determined microenvironment which regulates their fate and function. The surrounding ECM with its chemical and biophysical cues is a key element, so the lack of cell-ECM interaction limits their survival [73]. To try to overcome the problems of cells supply, alternative approaches are considered in current studies. The use of natural or synthetic materials in an injectable format, alone or together with cells (figure 1 b), has been investigated to limit remodeling and improve both cell attachment and survival upon implantation in the heart. Ideally, they should be tailored to be amenable to delivery with minimally invasive catheter based procedures [69]. The injectable materials have to cure or self-assemble rapidly (without the need or the release of toxic components) once delivered in the site of interest. As injected, they adopt the shape of the cavity, and may increase the stiffness and thickness of the ventricular wall [74]. Simulations showed that the injection of non-contractile materials with proper mechanical properties can contribute to limit the stress the ventricular wall withstands, thus helping to limit the remodeling [75].

These materials can help to keep the cells in the site of interest, provide them a 3D environment and also protect them from the hostile environment represented by the cytokines and hypoxic conditions, reactive oxygen species, etc., consequence of the infarcted condition of the site [41]. The injected gels can provide a cell friendly environment that will prevent anoikis [69]; they can also include adhesion motifs and then actively contribute to cell attachment. Moreover, they can be used as a controlled release system providing in a sustained way drugs or growth factors to improve cells survival, integration and proliferation [32]. And in the case of bioactive materials, their degradation products may provide additional chemicals that stimulate cells.

Among others, the ideal injectable material should be biodegradable, have a low immuno-genity, be no cytotoxic, non-adhesive and have antithrombogenic properties, adequate mechanical properties, provide stiffness to the scar but at the same time being compliant with the heart beating and transmit properly the mechanical stimuli to the cells, induce angiogenesis or at least not disturb the angiogenic activity after incorporation, be capable of delivering cells and or bioactive molecules [76]. Next, some of the materials investigated for their potential use as injectable ones are described.

4.2. *In situ* gelling biomaterials employed

4.2.1. Natural materials

Fibrin

Fibrin is a natural biopolymer that forms the natural provisory matrix for wound healing. It is FDA approved for many applications and there are different preparations commercially available, but it can also be obtained from autologous origin [77]; it is biocompatible, not toxic, or inflammatory [78]. Besides, some of the degradation products of fibrin have interesting properties, like improving healing promotion or a protective effect against myocardial reperfusion injury [79]. Fibrin contains arginine-glycine-asparagine (RGD), which are known cell adhesion motifs [77]; it is cytoprotective for anoxia and provides a favorable microenvironment for cardiomyogenic differentiation of marrow-derived cardiac stem cells [77]. It can also be used as a controlled release system [80]. In sum, fibrin as a gel is a potential candidate to enhance cell adhesion and survival. To obtain the fibrin, fibrinogen monomers in saline solution are mixed with thrombin and they polymerize forming a 3D net by mechanisms similar to normal clotting *in vivo* [81]. The properties of the network can be tailored by modifying the polymerization process.

A concern about translating the fibrin glue for cardiac tissue engineering into the clinic is the risk of inducing intravascular thrombosis [79]. The concentrations of fibrin amenable to delivery through current percutaneous catheters have been studied, demonstrating the feasibility of using fibrin in a non-invasive injectable application [81]. The injection of fibrin alone was proved to preserve left ventricular geometry and cardiac function in a rat acute MI model [82]. But it has also been combined with many types of cells. As an example, it was employed to deliver bone-marrow derived mesenchymal stem cells, which enhanced cell retention and prevented their redistribution in other organs, improving the beneficial effects of the treatment [81]. Injection of fibrin combined with myoblasts [82], bone marrow stem cells [83] or with autologous endothelial cells [84], improved the results obtained with cells alone.

Chitosan

Chitosan (CHT) is a natural cationic polysaccharide, obtained from the deacetylation of chitin of the mollusks, crustaceans and insects. It is soluble in acidic aqueous solution but after neutralization forms a gel-like precipitate [85]. CHT exhibits numerous positive biological and physicochemical properties: biocompatibility, non immunogenicity, and can be conjugated with various molecules thanks to the amino groups on the polysaccharide backbone [86]. A thermally responsive chitosan-based polymer was capable of scavenging the reactive oxygen species produced by the ischemic conditions and recruit key chemokines for stem cell homing such as SDF-1. As a cell delivery system with adipose-derived mesenchymal stem cells, this material was capable of improving the microenvironment for the cells when injected in the infarcted myocardium of rats, improving their survival and engraftment [87]. Chitosan mixed with collagen has been conjugated with QHREDGS (peptide thought to mediate attachment and survival responses of cardiomyocytes) in the format of a thermoresponsive hydrogel to improve maturation and metabolic activity of cardiomyocytes [86]. Alginate-chitosan nano-particles have been loaded with placental growth factor (PlGF) to increase the left-ventricular function and vascular density in rats [88].

Matrigel

Matrigel is a commercial ECM proteins mixture that undergoes a temperature mediated sol-gel transition, and is obtained from the ECM of mouse sarcoma cells [27]; its clinical application is limited precisely by the source from which it is obtained. It has been implanted alone and in combination with mouse ESC [89] or neonatal cardiomyocytes [90] into a mice model of infarcted myocardium. The gel prevented worsening of the cardiac function, but animals receiving both Matrigel and cells maintained more wall thickness and preserved better cardiac function in terms of fractional shortening and regional contractility [91].

Hair keratin

Keratin materials can be obtained from hair, importantly from autologous source. More than 30 growth factors are involved in hair morphogenesis, and the residual of them remains in the keratin, what can be beneficial for cardiac repair. Lyophilized keratin powders have the ability to self-assemble upon addition of water, and form gels. Keratin has been implanted onto infarcted rat hearts, and native cardiomyocytes as well as endothelial cells were able to infiltrate the keratin gel, promoting angiogenesis without inducing inflammation; after 2 months animals exhibited preservation of cardiac function and limited ventricular remodeling [92]. These improvements were attributed to the biomaterial's contribution to the mechanical support to the ventricular wall and the presence of cell binding motifs in it.

Alginate

Alginate is a linear block co-polymer of (1-4)-linked β-D-mannuronate and α-L-guluronate residues obtained from seaweed. It is a negatively charged polysaccharide that gels by the presence of calcium ions and is non-thrombogenic [4] The properties of this material can be tuned either by changing the concentration of the solutions or by controlling the molecular weight. Greater concentrations will increase mechanical strength but also will increase the solution viscosity and the degradation time of the gel [27].

Alginate has been used as an injectable material in recent and old infarcts in rats, and it was observed that its injection augmented the scar thickness and limited systolic and diastolic dysfunction [93]. It has also been proposed as a controlled delivery system: based on the different binding affinity of alginate to insulin-like growth factor-1 IGF-1 and hepatocyte growth factor HGF, a dual delivery system of these factors was developed [94]. The hydrogel beads protected the proteins from degradation maintaining their bioactivity and increasing the therapeutic effect of the system.

Alginate sustains very low protein adsorption and it does not support mammalian cells attachment [95], but it can be combined with adhesion motifs to improve its attachment properties. Its conjugation with RGD increased the arteriole density in a rodent model of chronic ischemic cardiomyopathy [96]. However, the combination of alginate with RGD and tyrosine–isoleucine– glycine–serine–arginine (YIGSR) reduced the therapeutic effects of the hydrogel in terms of scar thickness, left ventricular dilation and function [97]. Another modification of alginate has been the addition of the electrical conducting polymer polypyrrole [98], which increases arteriogenesis and promotes myofibroblasts infiltration.

Hyaluronic acid

Hyaluronic acid (HA) is a non-sulfated glycosaminoglycan prevalent in the extracellular matrix of many tissues. HA plays an important role in homeostasis, transport of nutrients and also mediates the inflammation and repair processes. It is biocompatible, non-immunogenic, biodegradable and has different biological activities depending on its molecular weight. Precisely the low molecular weight degradation products of HA stimulate angiogenesis and endothelial cell proliferation and migration [99]. It can be functionalized to improve its biological development, for example with PEG-SH$_4$ [100]. Moreover, it is a FDA-approved material for its use in humans in certain applications like dermal and intra-articular injection.

There are already commercially available *in situ* crosslinkable HA-derived hydrogels. Different types of HA hydrogels have been compared with commercial fibrin, poly(vinyl alcohol)-chitosan and elastin hydrogels, in terms of *in vitro* degradation rates and cytotoxicity and *in vivo* degradation, immune response and angiogenic potential [76]. Traut's grafted HA hydrogel and periodate oxidated HA hydrogel, especially the first one, demonstrated to be the most suitable for new artery formation in ischemic myocardium because they were both digested within 2 weeks with low immune response and strong angiogenesis compared with the other examined hydrogels.

HA alone does not support cell adhesion. Cardiosphere-derived cells were delivered using a thiolated hyaluronan-based hydrogel crosslinked with thiol-reactive poly(ethylene glycol) diacrylate and covalently linked or not with thiolated denatured collagen. It was observed that the retention rate achieved with the hydrogel without collagen was similar to that of cells delivered in phosphate buffer saline (PBS), either by a low physical retention or poor cell survival and adhesion of HA [101]. In the *in vivo* study in a mouse model of myocardial infarction, some functional benefits were observed though.

Collagen

Collagen supports growth and survival of cardiomyocytes *in vitro*, and is one of the main components of the ECM in the adult heart [102]. Commercial collagen alone has been implanted in animal models showing improvements in ventricular cardiac function and geometry [103]. In another study in a myocardial infarction model in rats (with ischemia-reperfusion model this time) increased capillarity density and myofibroblasts infiltration after 5 weeks were reported [104].

The therapeutic potential of injectable collagen has been evaluated in combination with different cell types. Bone marrow stem cells were injected via catheter in a swine model in combination with collagen, demonstrating the feasibility of a non-invasive delivery of this system [105]. Collagen was also used as a carrier for mesenchymal stem cells (MSC) transplantation to improve the retention of the cells in the infarcted myocardium [106]. 4

weeks after implantation, rats receiving cells in saline suspension, had the implanted cells in remote organs, whereas in animals receiving the cells with collagen, were detected to a lesser extent in remote organs. However, cardiac function was improved in animals receiving cells in saline and collagen alone but not in the combined collagen MSC group. The mechanisms underlying this negative interaction (controverted in other works) are unknown, but is suggested that collagen may limit oxygen and nutrients diffusion, and compromise cell-cell interactions. In another study, collagen combined with chondroitin 6-sulfate was employed to deliver CD-133+ progenitor cells derived from peripherial blood after expansion *in vitro* [107]. It was expected that the material would improve cell adhesion and survival into ischemic hind limb athymic rats. The collagen increased two-fold the number of cells retained when implanted alone; the implanted material was vascularized and the injected cells added into vascular structures.

Gelatin

It is a non-immunogenic partially degraded product of collagen [108]. It has been injected as a hydrogel in rat infarcted hearts bare or loaded with basic fibroblast growth factor; adding the factor improved arteriogenesis, ventricular remodeling and function [109]. Basic fibroblast growth factor has also been delivered with gelatin microspheres [110], inducing angiogenesis and improving cardiac function. The loaded nanoparticles induced an increase in the blood flow in the infarct border (thanks to stimulated angiogenesis), and as a result left ventricular function was improved.

ECM-derived materials

A different approach is based on decellularized tissues, their digestion and injection. This type of materials has the advantage of containing a physiological proportion of the native components of the ECM [102] and cues for cell-matrix interactions. ECM coming from different tissues has been studied, and apparently the ECM of each tissue has its unique combination of proteins and proteoglycans. This makes of myocardial decellularized matrix, among all other tissues matrices, the best candidate for myocardial repair when it is available [111]. Decellularized porcine myocardial tissue able to self-assemble into a nanofibrous structure similar to collagen *in vitro* at 37°C and deliverable *in vivo* upon catheter injection was tested in rats. It induced endothelial cells and smooth muscle cells migration increasing the arteriole formation at 11 days post-injection [111].

Small intestinal submucosa (SIS) is a dense sheet of acellular extracellular matrix. This material is used in the clinic for accelerated wound healing. SIS supports proliferation, attachment and migration of various cell types and stimulates angiogenesis thanks to the growth factors and binding motifs embedded in the matrix. Two different types of commercial available SIS-derived gels have been studied as an injectable material for cardiac repair in a murine model [112]. The two materials differed in the concentration of basic fibroblast factor, obtaining best result the material richer in this factor. In another work, an emulsion of digested ECM from SIS was injected into infarcted rat hearts, improving cardiac function, increasing neovascularization and promoting cell recruitment [113].

4.2.2. Synthetic materials

Synthetic materials are made in the laboratory from primary building blocks, so their properties can be tuned to match desired characteristics. Besides, they are free from animal origin components and the risks related therewith.

Thermosensitive hydrogels

This group of materials has temperature-dependant sol to gel transition. The great advantage of this group of materials is the possibility to tune their properties for them to undergo the gelation transition around body temperature [114]. In this way they can be comfortably manipulated and injected and only when they are inside the body they will undergo the transition.

Some of the materials of this group are based on N-isopropylacrylamide (NiPAAm). It is non biodegradable, but copolymerized with degradable polymers becomes biodegradable. For instance, NiPAAm was copolymerized with acrylic acid (AAc) and hydroxyethyl methacrylate-poly(trimethylene carbonate) (HEMAPTMC) [115]. The ratio of each material was adjusted to obtain a hydrogel at 37ºC. It can also be degraded *in vitro* with a mass loss over 85% after 5 months. This material was injected *in vivo* in rats and proved to preserve the area of the left ventricular cavity and contractility. Tissue ingrowth, a thicker left ventricle (LV) wall and greater capillarity density were also found when compared with PBS controls. After 8 weeks, a layer of smooth muscle cells with contractile phenotype was formed next to the remaining material.

Another family of thermoresponsive hydrogels based on polycaprolactone, N-isopropylacrylamide, 2-hydroxyethyl methacrylate and dimethyl-g-butyrolactone acrylate has been developed [116]. Cardiosphere derived cells (CDC) combined with the hydrogel were suitable for myocardial injection and the solutions formed solid gels within 5 s at 37ºC. Hydrogels with different mechanical properties were obtained and it was shown that they influence the fate of the CDC differentiation. Another thermoresponsive material containing biodegradable dextran chain grafted with hydrophobic poly(ε-caprolactone)-2-hydroxylethyl methacrylate (PCL-HEMA) chain and thermoresponsive poly(N isopropylacrylamide) (PNIPAAm) (Dex-PCL-HEMA/PNIPAAm) has been synthesized. It can shift from sol to gel within 30 s and is reversible within the same time frame [117]. It was injected in rabbits, 4-days post-infarction. Histological analyses one month later indicated that the material prevented the scar expansion and thinning of the wall. Left ventricular ejection fraction was increased and it attenuated left ventricular systolic and diastolic dilation.

Poly (Ethylene Glycol) (PEG)

A strategy based on non-biodegradable *in situ* crosslinkable PEG hydrogel has been developed, to provide a permanent support to limit the remodeling [118]. Its therapeutic effects were tested in rat myocardial infarction model at short and long term. Beneficial effects were observed at 4 weeks, but at long term (13 weeks) it was unable to prevent the dilation. Besides, the material injection induced some inflammatory response.

An injectable α-cyclodextrin/poly(ethylene glycol)–b-polycaprolactone-(dodecanedioic acid)-polycaprolactone–poly(ethylene glycol) (MPEG–PCL–MPEG) hydrogel was used to deliver and encapsulate bone marrow stem cells into infarcted myocardium [119]. The CD/MPEG-PCL-MPEG hydrogel alone does not induce angiogenesis, but can serve as a support in the infarcted zone and contribute to inhibit the left ventricular remodeling. One month after the injection of the gel combined with cells, cell retention and survival and the density of vessels were increased when compared with cells injection alone; moreover, the gel was absorbed, ventricular dilation was limited and the ventricular ejection fraction improved.

PEG-based temperature-sensitive hydrogels have also been combined with growth factors or other molecules. VEGF was mixed or conjugated with the aliphatic polyester hydrogel poly(δ-valerolactone)-block-poly(ethylene glycol)-block-poly(δ-valerolactone) (PVL-b-PEG-b-PVL); the sustained VEGF release during the degradation time of the hydrogel translated into an improvement of the myocardial and functional recovery, in dependence of the preparation method [120]. In another work, a metalloproteinase-responsive PEG-based hydrogel was synthesized to be a thymosin β4 (a pro-angiogenic and pro-survival factor) delivering scaffold. It was implanted combined with endothelial and smooth muscle cells derived from human embryonic stem cells (hESC) in rats [121]. The gel provides structural organization and when was loaded with cells and thymosin b4 enhanced more contractile performance than when the hydrogel was only loaded with the factor, because of their paracrine effect. Another PEG-based hydrogel, α-cyclodextrin/MPEG–PCL–MPEG, was tested as a delivery system for erythro-poietin (EPO) [122], a hormone that plays a protective role in the infarcted myocardium. Rats treated with this system showed limited cell apoptosis and increased neovasculature forma-tion; also infarct size was reduced and cardiac function improved.

PEG in the format of nanoparticles has also been studied. They can be injected intravenously, circulate in the body for long periods and bind only to desired tissues. Nanoparticles targeting the infarcted myocardium were developed based on the overexpression of angiotensin II type 1 (AT1) receptor in the infarcted heart [123]. The system was formed by a vehicle and a targeter, a ligand specific to AT1 that will make the nanoparticles bind specifically. The vehicle was 142 nm diameter PEGylated liposomes, which could carry therapeutic molecules and release them in a controlled way. This system was proved to target the infarcted heart in mice model, but not the healthy.

Self Assembling Peptides (SAPs)

SAPs are short peptides capable of forming hydrogels at physiological pH and osmolarity [124]. When the SAPs solution is placed in contact with ions or pH is changed, the charges are partially neutralized and a hydrophobic packing takes place forming beta-sheet structures, constituting fibers that build a 3D network if the concentration is high enough. Fibers shape is different depending on the nature of the employed peptides. In the particular case of the RAD16 ionic peptides family (R: arginine, A: alanine, D: aspartate) fibers thicknesses are of 5-10 nm.

Peptides can be combined with cells to encapsulate them within the peptide network [125]. RAD16-I (AcN-RADARADARADARADA-CNH$_2$) has proved to be a useful synthetic gel capable of maintaining the cells in the site of interest, and has been used as a delivery system of different types of cells to the heart. On the contrary, when it was implanted alone limited improvements were observed in the infarct area and the remodeling process. RAD16-II (AcN-RARADADARARADADA-CNH2) peptide has been shown to create microenvironments in the infarcted myocardium that are infiltrated with endothelial and smooth muscle cells, suggesting a potential for vascularization [124]. It was also observed that combining RAD16-II with neonatal cardiomyocytes the density of endogenous α-sarcomeric actin positive cells increased.

As stated, SAPs gels can be modified to incorporate growth factors or drugs. The self assembling peptide RAD16-II has been used as a drug vehicle to deliver both platelet derived growth factor and fibroblast growth factor (PDGF-BB and FGF-2) [126]. The first is arteriogenic and the second is angiogenic; their combination targets endothelial cells (EC) and vascular smooth muscle cells (VSMC). Infarct size and cardiomyocyte apoptosis were considerably reduced in rats. The capillary and arterial density was recovered, and cardiac function was almost recovered. This system also induced long-lasting vessel formation. RAD16-II combined with IGF-1, a cytokine that protects and promotes cardiomyocytes growth, has also been used as a delivery system for cardiomyocytes [127]. The addition of IGF-1 acted reducing cell apoptosis and improving systolic function.

5. Preformed gels and scaffolds

5.1. Rationale

An alternative approach in the field of cardiac tissue engineering involves the use of biomaterials to produce patches *ex vivo* and implant them epicardially onto the infarcted tissue, conveniently adapted to its size and shape. These patches can be pre-loaded with cells (incorporated within their pores in the case of microporous scaffolds, or encapsulated in the case of a gel conformed before implantation, as shown in figure 1 b) and growth factors or drugs, and act as a cell supply, a mechanical reinforcement to the infarct scar to avoid ventricular dilation and a drug release system simultaneously.

5.2. Requirements of the scaffolds

In this strategy a key aspect is to find a material that matches the required properties. The material needs also to be cell-friendly, non-cytotoxic and promote cell attachment and proliferation, and it must also be non-immunogenic [128]. The scaffolds should provide a 3D environment to the cells with a porous structure able to guide cardiomyocytes alignment and promote maturation, also induce the development of a contractile phenotype and the electro-mechanical coupling of the implanted cells among them, and also with the host tissue [129, 32] and need to be easily vascularized [37].

The mechanical properties exhibited by the scaffolds should be adequate to their application in heart tissue engineering. It implies that they should ideally be compliant with contractions and exhibit non-linear elasticity, as well as be capable to adapt to the shape of the heart in all phases of the heart beat. Anisotropy to mimic the directionally-dependent electrical and mechanical properties of the native myocardium is important too [130]. Besides, the stiffness of the material employed affects to a great extent the phenotype and contractile properties of the neonatal cardiomyocytes [131, 132], and has to be carefully tuned to match physiological conditions. During heart development, the ECM on which cardiomyocytes maturation takes place, stiffen 9 times. An interesting approach to mimic it is the development of materials with time dependant mechanical properties [133]. For instance, hyaluronic acid hydrogels that stiffen with time form more contractile units when compared with cultures in hydrogels without such time-dependant stiffness.

Attending to the type of strategy, three groups can be distinguished, in terms of the nature of the matrices: biologically-derived materials, synthetic (either biodegradable or biostable) materials and decellularized tissues. With the use of biodegradable scaffolds, it is expected that the matrix will degrade as the surrounding tissue is regenerated; the degradation products should not be toxic and metabolized by the body. By using permanent scaffolds, the idea is that they will be infiltrated by the host tissue and contribute to the regeneration, but also act as a permanent mechanical restraint to limit ventricular dilation. The approach of scaffolds derived from decellularized tissue is based on the use of tissues whose cells are removed and the remaining ECM maintains the architecture and mechanical properties similar to those of the native tissue. Obtaining a scaffold matching the desired properties is a hard task, as many different properties are required; thus, materials exhibiting different properties have been mixed in more advanced strategies to obtain a composite that combines them.

5.3. Related problematic

As all the approaches described so far, this one also has some advantages, disadvantages and unsolved problematic. An important disadvantage is that the application of a patch in the heart needs a much more invasive technique than a catheter-delivered system, as it requires a surgical procedure to be implanted. As advantage, the fact that the materials are synthesized and conveniently prepared out of the body can be outlined. It implies that there is no limitation in the preparation procedure and in the use of solvents (if they are properly removed at the end of the fabrication process and do not induce cytotoxicity). Therefore, the range of chemistries and techniques available to obtain scaffolds with different architectures is broadening. Besides, cells can be pre-cultured *in vitro* within them prior to implantation if desired. In addition, the mechanical properties of polymer scaffolds may be tuned to match more closely those of the heart muscle than with gelly biomaterials.

Unlike native myocardium, where the greatest distance between capillaries is around 20 microns [69], scaffolds are not vascularized *a priori*. Then, cells seeded in the scaffolds have their oxygen and nutrients supply limited to their molecular diffusion through the thickness of the scaffold. Given the fact that cardiomyocytes have great consumption rates of nutrients and oxygen, diffusion is insufficient supply for thick constructs. Consequently, to obtain a thick engineered tissue with viable cells through all its thickness, pre-vascularization or improved diffusion throughout the scaffold until it is vascularized is key for the implant to succeed. Otherwise, cell density will be concentrated in the external parts and cell viability will be compromised in the center of the scaffold if the distance to the surface is greater than a critical value estimated around 100 microns [134]. For example, the influence of oxygen concentration in cell density and viability in collagen scaffolds has been studied, the former decreasing linearly with the distance to the surface and the latter exponentially [135]. These results indicate that in order to guarantee an appropriate oxygen concentration throughout the scaffold, additional measures need to be taken.

Many attempts have been done in this direction, like the addition of oxygen carriers to the culture medium to simulate the effect of the hemoglobin in the blood. Their addition contributed to improve mass transport and to increase cell density [136]. Another strategy includes the use of scaffolds releasing growth factors to enhance the vascularization process, like basic fibroblast growth factor [137], vascular endothelial growth factor (VEGF) [138] and Thymosin beta-4 [139]. Another approach is the addition of the growth factor platelet derived growth factor BB to the culture medium to protect cardiomyocytes from apoptosis [140]. In a different methodology, channeled scaffolds were produced to simulate the capillary structure of the native tissues and guide endothelial cells growth. The porosity might be adjusted to increase capillary infiltration but it is limited to the maximum size of the pores on which endothelial cells can form vascular structures [141]. An alternative involves the use of decellularized tissues that already provide a native vascular network [142, 143]. The culture of endothelial cells prior to implantation of cardiac myocytes has also been explored [144], and reduced cardiomyocytes apoptosis and necrosis was found. Another possibility is to pre-implant the scaffold to pre-vascularize it prior to its implantation in the final site: alginate scaffolds loaded with angiogenic and pro-survival factors (Matrigel, SDF-1, VEGF and IGF-1) were pre-implanted into the omentum of rats [145]. It proved to be a very interesting *in vivo* "bioreactor", providing to the patch a functional vascular network that maintained the viability of the transplanted cells.

Pre-culturing the scaffolds *in vitro* in bioreactors has also been a considered an option. There are many types of bioreactors (stirring, spinning flasks rotating, perfusion, etc.), but not all of them improve enough the diffusion to lead to uniform cell density and compact tissue formation. As an example, in a study where rotating bioreactors were used to culture poly-glycolic acid (PGA) scaffolds [146], functional and interconnected cells only were found in the peripheral parts, where there was a better diffusion of the oxygen. Perfusion bioreactors have been developed to try to reduce diffusional limitations by establishing interstitial flow through the scaffolds in order to allow the formation of thick tissues with uniform cell density throughout them. The effect of culturing scaffolds in perfusion bioreactors was compared with culturing them in spinner flasks [134] or orbital mixed dishes [147]. In both studies results were improved with the perfusion bioreactors; when cultured in the others, high cell density was only found in the outer layers. However, a limitation of perfusion bioreactors is the medium flow rate, because of the hydrodynamic shear the interstitial flow inflicts to the cells, which could maintain them in a rounded morphology or even wash them out if it is too high. This finding led to the combination of the perfusion culture with the use of channeled scaffolds that provided separated compartments for medium flow [148]. Even more, this strategy has been successfully combined and used simultaneously with a selective pre-seeding of the scaffold in the channels with endothelial cells using a perfusion seeding technique, which provides uniform seeding throughout the entire scaffold without the use of cell carriers [149].

Another step was made when the pulsatile perfusion bioreactor [150] was developed. It was expected that the pulsatile interstitial medium flow would provide mechanical conditioning and improved mass transport, intending that all together would lead to a tissue with better contractile properties. Indeed, scaffolds cultured under these conditions had enhanced contractile properties. A different type of bioreactor, with bidirectional slow flow perfusion obtained with an oscillatory system was tested with culture medium loaded or not with Insuline-like growth factor-I [151]. The advantage of the combined strategies was revealed.

However, despite the great efforts put and the improvements achieved, obtaining vascularized constructs is still an unsolved problem.

5.4. Preparation techniques

Many different techniques have been proposed to obtain 3D porous structures with different topographies and porosities, basically based in phase separation procedures or the use porogen templates to create the pores. Now with the introduction of controlled computer assisted systems, new possibilities are open. Next, a brief description of the main techniques employed to prepare scaffolds for heart tissue engineering is outlined.

The electrospinning technique is based in the application of a high voltage to a polymer melted or in a solution that leads to the formation of ultrathin nonwoven fibers [152], which are projected on a collector giving rise to fiber mats with controlled thicknesses. The fibers diameters can be obtained in the range of the ECM proteins. This technique also allows the preparation of aligned fibers, which can be applied to obtain aligned cardiac cells [153].

The particle leaching technique is based on the use of a porogen that is mixed with a polymer solution or a melted polymer. This porogen is removed after the solvent has been eliminated (solvent casting, freeze extraction) or the polymer has solidified after cooling, leaving empty spaces (pores) with the size and shape of the porogen template (and also small pores for the elimination of the solvent, if used). Porosity and pores interconnection can be tuned by changing the porogen-polymer ratio. Gas foaming avoids the use of solvents and high temperatures, because the pores are obtained by exposition to a high pressure gas followed by a pressure decrease with nucleation and growth of pores. The freeze-drying technique consists in freezing a polymeric solution and then lyophilize it to remove the solvent in the frozen state and obtain a solid porous structure [154]. Different morphologies can be obtained by changing the freezing conditions [155].

Microfluidic patterning consists in forcing a polymer solution through a channeled mould previously obtained with the desired geometry. Once the polymer is consistent, the mould is removed and the scaffold or patterned surface is ready. Selective laser sintering is a technique based in the use of a CO_2 laser to sinterize selectively the powder of a material to form the cross section of each layer of a 3D object.

Microcontact printing is a technique that allows cell adhesion guidance [156]. It consists in the use of a stamp, with the pattern to be followed by the cells. The stamp is inked with the solution that is expected to promote the adhesion (laminin, ECM proteins, etc.) and then pressed against the substrate to transfer the solution. By loading the solution with growth factors, cell differentiation can also be induced in patterns [157].

5.5. Biomaterials employed as scaffolds

Many different types of materials have been considered for cardiac tissue engineering. According to their origin we can distinguish: biologically-derived materials, decellularized tissues and synthetic materials. Natural materials include collagen, gelatin, fibrin, silk and alginate; and synthetic materials include polyurethane (PU), polylactide acid (PLA), polyglycolic acid (PGA), polycaprolactone (PCL), or polyglicerolsebacate (PGS), among others.

5.5.1. Natural materials

Collagen

There are a number of commercial collagen patches, widely used by clinicians for other purposes, which are now under study as epicardial patches, because it has been reported to be a good substrate for cell attachment and infiltration [158]. They have been combined with different cell types and molecules. Unfortunately, collagen sponges have a great swelling rate and poor mechanical performance in aqueous medium.

Collagen can be used in two formats, as a porous scaffold or as a hydrogel. To obtain the scaffold a collagen solution is lyophilized and then rehydrated and seeded with cells. In the case of hydrogels, a collagen solution is mixed with cells *ex vivo* and then gelled. As a gel entrapping embryonic chick cardiomyocytes [159], it was found to beat and arrange as a highly organized tissue-like when pulses with different frequency were applied.

The potential of collagen scaffolds as an attractant for neovascularization was demonstrated in a study with rats [160]. Collagen sponges implanted in both healthy and cryoinjured hearts were almost absorbed after 2 months, but the remaining structures were populated by new arterioles and capillaries. In another study, collagen has been combined with chondroitin 6-sulfate to obtain porous scaffolds. These scaffolds delivered MSC in the infarcted region in a rat model, promoting neovascularization [161].

The therapeutical potential of collagen as epicardial patch has been compared with injectable approaches. Collagen matrices loaded with mesenchymal stem cells (MSC) [162], and collagen scaffolds loaded with human umbilical cord blood cells (hUCBCs) [25], gave better results than the injection of cells alone in mice. In the MAGNUM phase I clinical trial [163], intrainfarct cell therapy of autologous BMC was combined with collagen scaffolds loaded with BMC. This treatment was found to be safe and contribute to limit left ventricular remodeling by increasing the thickness of the ventricle wall and then reducing the stress of the wall.

Collagen has been modified to incorporate bioactive molecules to improve its biological behavior. Its scaffolds have been modified with RGD [164] and cardiac markers of cardiospheres derived from cardiac progenitor cultured on them were upregulated. Collagen functionalized with interleukin-10 plasmid [165] (an anti-inflammatory plasmid) increased 5 times cell retention and modulated inflammation.

Gelatin

Gelatin is obtained from chemical denatured collagen; it is therefore weaker and degrades faster than it [27]. It has been reported to provoke unspecific inflammatory response upon degrading; at first this can be considered an undesired effect, but for certain applications it might be beneficial for the positive impact that can have on angiogenesis [166]. A commercial gelatin sponge bare or cultured either with fetal or adult rat heart cells was implanted to replace the resected right ventricular outflow tract (ROVT) of rats [167]. After 4 weeks a great inflammation was observed and after 12 weeks the patches had endothelial cells on the endocardial surface. Nonetheless, the authors concluded that a material inducing less inflammatory response is needed.

Fibrin

Fibrin can be used as an injectable gel, but can also be preformed *ex vivo*, which broadens the possibilities of fabrication. For example, SDF-1 (a factor that is up-regulated for a period of time after a myocardial infarction, and contributes to mobilize cells from bone marrow and peripherial blood to the damaged tissue) was covalently bound to a PEGylated fibrin patch [168] and implanted in an AMI mouse model; the SDF-1 loaded patch reduced more significantly the scar area expansion and improved the left ventricular function than the un-loaded patch.

Alginate

Alginate scaffolds obtained by the freeze drying technique have been extensively explored in myocardial regeneration. Loaded with fetal cardiac cells and implanted in infarcted rats, they limited left ventricular dilation [169]. However, cultured with neonatal or fetal cardiomyocytes in static conditions, cell aggregates were formed due to the nonadhesive nature of the alginate [170].

To improve cell adhesion and survival modifications of alginate scaffolds have been investigated. For example, it has been modified to incorporate the adhesion peptide RGD [171], which improved cell adhesion, reduced apoptosis, accelerated tissue regeneration and led to the organization of cardiomyocytes in myofibers *in vitro*, and also with a combination of RGD and the heparin-binding peptide G4SPPRRARVTY (HBP) [172], with better results.

Polysaccharides

Polysaccharide-based scaffolds have also been investigated with myocardial regeneration purposes. The effectiveness of freeze-dried pullulan and dextran patches was compared to mesenchymal stem cells endocardial delivery alone in a rat myocardial infarction model [173], the scaffolds improving the cell engraftment and survival at 1 and 2 months.

Silk

Because of silk fibroin good mechanical properties, biological performance, and its easy processing to obtain different morphologies, it has generated interest in the tissue engineering field. Silk is produced by some insects like spiders or silkworms, and is considered a non-degradable material by the FDA [174]. Silk fibroin has been combined by chitosan and hyaluronic acid to produce microparticles that were pressed and crosslinked with genipin to obtain cardiac patches [175]. MSC cultured on the composite patches exhibited greater proliferation and cardiomyogenic differentiation than in silk patches.

Recently, non-mulberry silk fibroin from Antheraea mylitta has been investigated as a material for cardiac tissue engineering [176]. It has better mechanical properties than mulberry silk, contains RGD sequences, is non-cytotoxic and induces low level of inflammatory response. When neonatal rat cardiomyocytes were seeded in an Antherea mylitta silk lyophilized scaffold, the results were better than those obtained with a mulberry silk.

Decellularized-tissue derived scaffolds

Decellularized extracellular matrices have been used as scaffolds in many studies and also in preclinical and human clinical applications [177]. The decellularization process consists in a set of washes to remove the cells but maintain as much as possible the architecture, proteins and adhesion molecules. The more aggressive the washes and treatments are, the lower the risk of allogenic immune reaction is, but undesired washout of adhesion proteins and architecture damage can be associated [65].

Decellularized sheets have been tested in combination with fibrin, TGF-beta, and MSC and tested in a nude rat model of infarction with positive results [178]. A patch of urinary bladder-derived extracellular matrix (UBM) was implanted in pigs, as a left ventricular wall replacement after infarction, and compared with a polytetrafluoroethlyene (ePTFE) [177] one. At three months, the results were better with the UBM: it was reabsorbed and a cellularized and vascularized tissue rich in collagen was formed.

Sliced decellularized porous scaffolds of acellular bovine pericardia have been combined with cell sheets from bone marrow stem cells, cultured and implanted in rats replacing the resected infarcted myocardium [179]. The patch pores were filled by cells, new vessels and new muscle fibers, indicating that the graft was integrating. Cardiac function was improved and the dilated left ventricle was restored after implantation. In a revolutionary study entire rat hearts were decellularized, and then re-cellularized with neonatal cardiac cells [180]. The architecture was conserved and the preserved vasculature was perfusable. Seeded cardiomyocytes coupled electromechanically and after 8 days under external electrodes stimulation the re-cellularized heart beat and was capable to pump blood.

5.5.2. Synthetic materials

Synthetic materials are prepared in the laboratory, allowing precise control over their mechanical properties, degradation, morphology and porosity that can be tuned as desired

[181]. However, they may not have as good biological performance as biologically derived materials [4].

Polylactic Acid and Polyglycolic Acid (PLA and PGA)

Polylactic acid is a biocompatible, biodegradable and FDA-approved polymer; it degrades into lactic acid (non-cytotoxic), and has been widely used in patients, for example as sutures. However, its degradation products can induce a slight, undesired, acidification of the microenvironment [65]. Polyglycolic acid is a thermoplastic too; it has also been used in the clinic and degrades into non-toxic products. However, neither PLLA nor PGA exhibit the desired elasticity to match that of native heart tissue. In many studies PLA and PGA have been combined as poly(lactic–co-glycolic acid) (PLGA), or other polyesters, to modify their properties as desired. Electrospun PLGA fibrous membranes with different compositions (having different hydrophobicity and degradation rates) [4] were found to align cardiomyocytes in the direction of the nanofibers, the best results being those of the slightly hydrophobic copolymers. Porous beads of PLGA seeded with human amniotic fluid stem cells (hAFSCs) have been tested as a cell delivery vehicle or "cellularized microscaffold" [182]; after implantation by intramyocardial injection in a rat infarct model, they showed good retention of the cells in the site of interest. PLGA has been treated with laminin [183] to improve its biological development and combined with carbon nanofibers (CNF) to increase its conductivity and cytocompatibility [184]. PLLA-PLGA scaffolds loaded with Matrigel have been co-cultured with endothelial cells, cardiomyocytes and embryonic fibroblasts simultaneously [185], for EC to provide vasculature and act synergically with cardiomyocytes to improve cell survival and proliferation.

Poly (epsilon-caprolactone) (PCL)

Poly(epsilon-caprolactone) is a FDA-approved biocompatible polyester, as PLA and PGA. It is more elastic because of its lower glass transition temperature, and behaves as a rubber at body temperature. Its degradation does not produce acidification because it occurs more slowly [158]. It has been proposed for myocardial regeneration for example in 3D constructs obtained by overlapping electrospun PCL nanofibrous mats (up to 5 layers) on which neonatal cardiomyocytes were cultured [186]. The layers established morphologic and electrical connections between them and exhibited synchronized beating, and no ischemia was found in the center of the constructs.

It is usually combined with PLA, PGA or its copolymer. Poly-glycolide-co-caprolactone (PGCL) biodegradable porous scaffolds have been studied as cell vehicles for bone marrow-derived mononuclear cells (BMMNC) in rat myocardial infarction models [187]. BMNC migrated from the scaffold and neovasculature over the implant was detected; left ventricular function improvement and limitation of the progression of the left ventricular dilation was also observed. Scaffolds made of poly(DL-lactide-*co*-caprolactone) (PLACL), PLGA, and type I collagen [158], cultured with neonatal rat heart cells, have been compared. The composite scaffolds gave better results than controls (collagen and PLGA sponges) in terms of cellularity, contractility and cardiac markers expression (Tn-I and Cx-43). Perfusion culture improved cell density distribution.

Polyurethanes (PU)

Polyurethanes are synthetic biocompatible materials widely used in the biomedical field. Their mechanical properties and biodegradability can be tuned by changing their composition. PU degrades *in vivo* through hydrolytic chain scission, which is accelerated by the enzymes action and loads, among other factors [188], but with the appropriate composition non-biodegradable polyurethanes can be obtained [189]. This family of polymers can be used to obtain fibrous scaffolds by electrospinning with different mechanical properties depending on the fibers orientation [190] or porous elastic scaffolds [191]. Polyester urethane urea (PEUU) elastic porous scaffolds have been implanted in sub-acute infarctions in rats and were found to promote the formation of smooth muscle bundles, to increase the ventricle thickness and to improve contractile function [192]. Cell attachment on polyurethane-based porous scaffolds can be improved by pre-treating them with laminin [193].

Poly(glycerol sebacate) (PGS)

Poly(glycerol sebacate) is a biocompatible and biodegradable elastomer capable of recovering from deformation. It can be obtained by polycondensation of glycerol and sebacic acid. By changing the synthesis temperature, the properties of the resulting material can be tuned to match the desired mechanical properties. The degradation rates can also be adjusted from fast degradation to nearly inert [194].

By the use of excimer laser microablation, 3D porous PGS scaffolds with anisotropic structural and mechanical properties were obtained [195, 130]. These scaffolds induced neonatal cardiac cells alignment in the absence of external stimuli and matched the mechanical properties of adult rat right ventricle. Moreover, they allowed cell contractility when stimulated. For its interesting mechanical properties, PGS has been coaxially electrospun with gelatin to form a nanofibrous mat with PGS in the core and gelatin in the shell [196] to enhance cell adhesion and proliferation. PGS has been modified to incorporate acrylic groups in different number (to modify its mechanical properties and degradation) and electrospun in combination with gelatin [197].

Acrylate based materials

Acrylate based materials have not been widely exploited for cardiac tissue engineering yet but the interest on them is increasing, for their versatility of processing and variety of properties obtained. For example, scaffolds made of poly(2-hydroxyethyl methacrylate-co-methacrylic acid) (P(HEMA-co-MAA) hydrogel have been obtained by fibers and microspheres templating to obtain spherical pores and parallel channels [198], which allow simultaneously mass transfer and guidance of the cardiomyocyte bundles. Mechanical properties were adjusted intentionally for the elastic modulus to be lower than that of native myocardium in order to make possible the mechanical stimulation of the cells when implanted *in vivo*. In [199], poly(ethyl acrylate) (PEA) scaffolds are filled with HA gel; the scaffolds provide the three-dimensional environment and mechanical properties and the gel may act as an encapsulating medium for the cells and may be also used as a medium for drug or growth factors release. RAD16-I gel may also be used as a filler in PEA scaffolds, where it acts as a diffusion medium and improves cell seeding efficiency (figure 2).

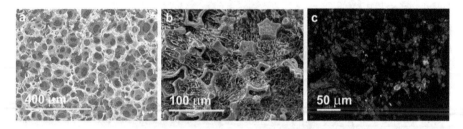

Figure 2. (a) Scanning electron microscopy (SEM) image of poly(ethyl acrylate), PEA, elastomeric membranes with interconnected spherical pores. (b) CryoSEM image (cross section) of a PEA scaffold whose pores are filled with the self-assembling peptide (SAP) gel RAD16-I. (c) Adipose stem cells (nuclei stained in blue and actin cytoskeleton stained in green) seeded in a PEA scaffold with a SAP gel filling. Confocal laser scanning microscopy image of a 50 μm thick internal slice.

5.6. Electrical and mechanical stimulation

Electrical stimulation

External electrical fields have been shown to contribute to the differentiation towards cardiomyocytes of different cell types, such as embryonic stem cells (ESC) [200] or BMSC [201] seeded in collagen scaffolds, and to the development of conductive and contractile properties of neonatal cardiac cells, in this case seeded with Matrigel in a collagen porous scaffold [202]. It has been proposed that the intracellular endogenous reactive oxygen species (ROS) produced when an electric field is applied contribute to the hESC differentiation [203].

In an attempt of optimizing the electrical stimulation parameters [204], it has been determined that the electrode material is very important, and best results have been obtained for carbon electrodes. Amplitude and frequency of the stimulation have also a great influence in the cultured cardiac tissue. Micropatterned electrodes can be of interest as they allow spatial control of the electric field [205].

Polymeric scaffolds limit cardiomyocytes electric communication, what restricts the synchronous beating of the engineered tissue. To improve it, gold nanowires were incorporated to a porous alginate scaffold [206]. Another approach to obtain elastic and electrical conductive scaffolds consisted in impregnating thiol-HEMA/HEMA scaffolds with gold nanoparticles [207]. In both cases even without electrical stimulation the improvement in the scaffold conductivity had positive physiological effects.

Mechanical stimulation

Mechanical stress has a great impact on cell proliferation, ECM formation and hypertrophy (increased cell size), and has been intensively studied in the field of cardiac tissue engineering. Embryonic chick and neonatal rat cardiac myocytes mixed with collagen and mechanically stimulated exhibited hypertrophy and improvement of contractile function [208]. Cardiac myocytes from neonatal rats mixed with collagen I and Matrigel and casted in rings subjected to mechanical stretch [209] showed histological characteristics of adult cardiac tissue. Action potential measurements indicated electrophysiological behavior akin to cardiac tissue.

Constructs produced by simultaneously electrospinning PU and electrospraying mesenchymal stem cells [210] were cultured in spinner flasks with stretching, which led to cells alignment, cardiac markers increase and ion channels development. Similarly, cells isolated from neonatal rat hearts seeded in chitosan-collagen I channeled porous scaffolds [211] and cultured under high mechanical stimulation induced cell alignment, elongation and the presence of gap junctions connecting the cells. Mechanical stress applied to human cardiac cells cultured in a gelatin scaffold improved cell distribution and proliferation within the scaffold, increased the production of the ECM, and the structure and organization was similar to normal myocardium, likely because the stretching of the scaffold favors nutrients and oxygen exchange improving cell microenvironment [212].

6. Ventricular restraints

After Chachques and Carpentier work [213], it was found that wrapping the heart even with a passive muscle flap had beneficial effects; this finding led to the development of the ventricular restraint therapy [214]. In this approach the aim is not to regenerate the ischemic tissue, but to avoid the progress of the adverse remodeling following a myocardial infarction. It is based on the application of a mechanical restraint (schematized in figure 1 c), which should limit or revert ventricular dilation. A variety of synthetic meshes have been proposed to achieve this goal.

A bilayer membrane with polypropylene in one side to promote tissue ingrowth (or at least limit the ventricular dilation) and with polytetrafluoroethylene in the other side to prevent pericardial adhesions was studied in a chronic infarction model of pig as a restraint [215]. The use of this patch induced improvements once the remodeling process following an infarction had started. The use of a non-biodegradable material is intentional as authors considered that a permanent mechanical reinforcement would be necessary to limit the remodeling.

To determine the extent at which a mechanical restraint is beneficial, a comparative study of two types of restrain was carried out in sheep: a patch over the infarct (non-biodegradable Marlex mesh) or a wrap (non-biodegradable Merseline mesh) [216]. The use of the mesh wrapping the ventricle reduced the remodeling whereas the patch applied over the infarct did not yield considerable improvements when compared with controls (untreated infarcted animals).

Paracor heartnet is a nitinol mesh proposed as a restrain device that is under clinical study in patients with severe dilated cardiomyopathy. In a study, six months after the implantation in 51 patients, results obtained suggested clinical benefits tending to reverse remodeling and that it could consequently be reliably implanted [217]. The PEERLESS-HF trial is the last carried out with this device so far [218]. It proved to be safe and improved patient's quality of life and ventricular dilation; however, no improvement in the peak of VO_2 was produced (which was an end-point of the trial), what led to stop enrollment in the trial. Nevertheless, a new clinical trial is planned. In another study in an animal model, it was shown that the heartnet can alter myocardial blood flow patterns in dilated cardiomyopathy, although it remains unclear if these changes are clinically relevant [219].

Another left ventricular restraint proposed is Acorn Corcap, a polyester mesh that is also being assessed in clinical trials after the positive results obtained in animal models [220]. 5 years after implantation it exhibited safety, a sustained reverse remodeling with a significant reduction in the left ventricular end diastolic volume and a slight increase in the sphericity index [221]. However, in an echocardiographic study using tissue velocity imaging, no improvement in cardiac output was achieved [222].

Limited results obtained with the ventricular restraint therapy can be, among other reasons, because of the absence of tissue regeneration. A more advanced approach combines the ventricular restraint therapy with a regenerative strategy such as patches or scaffolds loaded with cells. For instance, the Acorn Corcap and a collagen matrix loaded with MSC has been implanted in sheeps, and the combination was found to limit the fibrosis produced as foreign body reaction against the Corcap and improve the systolic and diastolic function [223].

7. Concluding remarks

Several therapeutic strategies have been proposed in the last decade to limit the adverse spread of the ischemic tissue and ventricle dilation or even to generate new myocardial tissue. These treatments consist in cellular therapy (so-called cellular cardiomyoplasty) where cells of different origin are implanted by different techniques onto the infarcted ventricle with the hope that cells will contribute to the generation of new contractile tissue to replace the scar, electrically coupled with the host myocardium. But despite the intense efforts and work put in the field, attempts so far have failed. Most of the implanted cells die soon after transplantation due to the fact that the cells cannot withstand the mechanical forces they experience in the host tissue. Mechanisms underlying the slight improvements observed are still undetermined; the paracrine effect is usually considered the way through which cells act, but the precise mechanisms are not completely understood yet. Besides, for this therapeutic approach to evolve to a realistic alternative to conventional treatments, some critical issues are still to be clarified: the way of delivery to maximize cell engraftment and minimize cell loss and death, the ideal cell type to be used, and the optimal time of cell administration (if they are implanted too soon, the inflammatory process kills the implanted cells, but if it is too late, the presence of the fibrotic scar limits their beneficial effects). New strategies already under study envision to improve cell survival by pre-conditioning the cells, pre-treating the host tissue or combining cells with other elements.

A possible way of localizing the appropriate cells in the target diseased tissue is to entrap them in a cell-friendly gelling biomaterial. Besides, gels can incorporate bioactive molecules for their controlled supply, and their preparation procedure (in the case of *in situ* gelling materials) avoids any invasive surgery. The injection of gelly materials alone onto the infarcted myocardium has shown some beneficial effects by itself and contributes somehow to limit the ventricular remodeling, for their slight role as mechanical support. Combining cells with gelly materials contributes, to some extent, to increase the cells residence time in the site of interest, and enhances cells adhesion and survival by providing them a better microenvironment. However, the consistency of these materials is generally too weak to withstand the synchronous contraction of the heart muscle without spreading from their target location, and their mechanical properties are too low to reach significant improvements in terms of containment of the dilated ventricle and post-infarct ventricular dysfunction.

Alternative tissue engineering strategies combine cells with three-dimensional scaffolds or patches to host them and improve their survival, induce the formation of new blood vessels and extracellular matrix and at the same time support the native tissue mechanically. The advantages of using myocardial patches or scaffolds are not only their usually superior mechanical properties, but also their wide versatility in terms of chemistries and morphology. There are many fabrication techniques for the preparation of scaffolds, leading to very different architectures, and these options are broadening with the computer-assisted techniques. Generally, positive results have been obtained by using scaffolds. In studies in which the therapeutic efficiency of a material was compared when used as an injectable gel or as a pre-fabricated scaffold or patch, the scaffold gave better results. When the scaffolds were loaded with growth factors or adhesion motives, in most of the cases the outcome was better. Mechanical and electrical stimulation are of help for cardiomyocytes to mature within the scaffolds and develop the characteristics and structures typical of cardiac tissue. Unfortunately, the implantation of epicardiac patches is much more invasive than that of injectable gels, and they need to be vascularized to ensure the success of the graft. Many attempts have addressed these questions but a satisfying solution has not been found yet.

Acknowledgements

The authors acknowledge the support of the FP7 NMP3-SL-2009-229239 project "Regeneration of cardiac tissue assisted by bioactive implants (RECATABI)".

Author details

M. Arnal-Pastor[1], J. C. Chachques[2], M. Monleón Pradas[1,3*] and A. Vallés-Lluch[1]

*Address all correspondence to: mmonleon@ter.upv.es

1 Center for Biomaterials and Tissue Engineering, Universitat Politècnica de València, Cno. de Vera s/n, Valencia, Spain

2 Department of Cardiovascular Surgery, Laboratory of Biosurgical Research, Georges Pompidou European Hospital, Paris, France

3 Networking Research Center on Bioengineering, Biomaterials and Nanomedicine (CIBER-BBN), Valencia, Spain

References

[1] Roger VL et al. Heart Disease and Stroke Statistics - 2012 Update A Report From the American Heart Association. Circulation 2012; 125: 2-220.

[2] Vasan SV, Benjamin EJ, Sullivan LM, D'agostino RB. The burden of increasing worldwide cardiovascular disease. In: Fuster V, Walsh RA, O'Rourke RA, Poole-Wilson P (ed.) Hurst the Heart. 12th edition McGraw-Hill Professional; 2010 p17-46.

[3] World Hearth Organition. WHO: Programes and projects: Cardiovascular disease: The Atlas of Heart Disease and Stroke; 2004. http://www.who.int/cardiovascular_diseases/resources/atlas/en/ (accessed 03 June 2012)

[4] Venugopal JR, Prabhakaran MP, Mukherjee S, Ravichandran R, Dan K, Ramakrishna S. Biomaterial Strategies for Alleviation of Myocardial Infarction. Journal of the Royal Society Interface 2012; 9(66): 1-19. doi:10.1098/rsif.2011.0301.

[5] Walker CA, Spinale FG. The Structure and Function of the Cardiac Myocite: a Review of Fundamental Concepts. The Journal of Thoracic and Cardiovascular Surgery 1999; 118: 375-82.

[6] Di Donato M, Toso A, Dor V, Sabatier M, Barletta G, Menicanti L, Fantini F and the RESTORE Group. Surgical Ventricular Restoration Improves Mechanical Intraventricular Dyssynchrony in Ischemic Cardiomyopathy. Circulation 2004; 109: 2536-43.

[7] Smaill BH, LeGrice IJ, Hooks DA, Pullan AJ, Caldwell BJ, Hunter PJ. Cardiac Structure and Electrical Activation: Models and Measurement. Clinical and Experimental Pharmacology and Physiology 2004; 31 (12): 913-9.

[8] Kocica MJ, Corno AF, Carreras-Costa F, Ballester-Rodes M, Moghbel MC, Cueva CNC, Lackovic V, Kanjuh V, Torrent-Guasp F. The Helical Ventricular Myocardial Band: Global, Three-Dimensional, Functional Architecture of the Ventricular Myocardium. European Journal Cardio-Thoracic Surgery 2006; 29: 21-40. DOI: 10.1016/j.ejcts.2006.03.011

[9] LeGrice IJ, Smaill BH, Chai LZ, Edgar SG, Gavin JB, Hunter PJ. Laminar Structure of the Heart: Ventricular Myocyte Arrangement and Connective Tissue Architecture in the Dog. American Journal of Physiology 1995; 269: H571-82.

[10] Chen FY, Cohn LH. The Surgical Treatment of Heart Failure. A New Frontier: Non-transplant Surgical Alternatives in Heart Failure. Cardiology in Review 2002; 10(6): 326-33.

[11] Hoyt RH, Cohen ML, Saffitz JE. Distribution and Three-Dimensional Structure of Intercellular Junctions in Canine Myocardium. Circulation Research 1989; 64: 563-74.

[12] Spach MS, Heidlage JF. The Stochastic Nature of Cardiac Propagation at a Microscopic Level. Electrical Description of Myocardial Architecture and its Application to Conduction. Circulation Research 1995; 76: 366-80.

[13] Severs NJ. The Cardiac Muscle Cell. BioEssays 2000; 22: 188-199.

[14] Burke AP, Virmani R. Pathology of myocardial ischemia, infarction, reperfusion and sudden death. In: Fuster V, Walsh RA, O'Rourke RA, Poole-Wilson P (ed.) Hurst the Heart. 12th edition McGraw-Hill Professional; 2010. p1321-1338.

[15] Baig MK, Mahon N, McKenna WJ, Caforio ALP, Bonow RO, Francis GS, Gheorghiade M. The Pathophysiology of Advanced Heart Failure. Heart & Lung 1999; 28(2): 87-101.

[16] Ferrero JM Jr, Trénor B, Montilla F, Saiz J, Ferrero Á, Rodriguez B. Ischemia. In: Wiley Encyclopedia of Biomedical Engineering. (ed.) John Wiley & Sons, Inc; 2006. p1-17.

[17] Douglas JS Jr, King SB III.Percutaneous coronary intervention. In:. Fuster V, Walsh RA, O'Rourke RA, Poole-Wilson P (ed.) Hurst the Heart. 12th edition McGraw-Hill Professional; 2010. p1427-1457.

[18] Lally C. Kelly DJ, Prendergast PJ. Stents. In: Wiley Encyclopedia of Biomedical Engineering. (ed.) John Wiley & Sons, Inc; 2006. p1-10.

[19] Stefanini GG, Kalesan B, Serruys PW, Heg D, Buszman P, Linke A, Ischinger T, Klauss V, Eberli F, Wijns W, Morice MC, Di Mario C, Corti R, Antoni D, Sohn HY, Eerdmans P, van Es GA, Meier B, Windecker S, Jüni P. Long-term clinical outcomes of biodegradable polymer biolimus-eluting stents versus durable polymer sirolimus-eluting stents in patients with coronary artery disease (LEADERS): 4 year follow-up of a randomised non-inferiority trial. Lancet 2011; 378: 1940-8.

[20] Ruwende C, Visovatti S, Pinsky DJ. Molecular and cellular mechanisms of myocardial ischemia-reperfusion injury. In: Fuster V, Walsh RA, O'Rourke RA, Poole-Wilson P (ed.) Hurst the Heart. 12th edition McGraw-Hill Professional; 2010. p1339-1350.

[21] Nian M, Lee P, Khaper N, Liu P. Inflammatory Cytokines and Postmyocardial Infarction Remodeling. Circulation Research 2004; 94: 1543-1553.

[22] Sun Y, Kiani MF, Postlethwaite AE, Weber KT. Infarct Scar as Living Tissue. Basic Research in Cardiology 2002; 97: 343-347. doi: 10.1007/s00395-002-0365-8.

[23] Christman KL, Lee RJ. Biomaterials For the Treatment of Myocardial Infarction. Journal American College of Cardiology 2006; 48: 907-13.

[24] Mann DL. Mechanisms and Models in Heart Failure: a Combinatorial Approach. Circulation 1999; 100: 999-1008. DOI: 10.1161/01.CIR.100.9.999.

[25] Cortes-Morichetti M, Frati G, Schussler O, Duong Van Huyen JP, Lauret E, Genovese JA, Carpentier AF, Chachques JC. Association Between a Cell-Seeded Collagen Ma-

trix and Cellular Cardiomyoplasty for Myocardial Support and Regeneration. Tissue engineering 2007; 13(11): 2681-2687. doi: 10.1089/ten.2006.0447.

[26] Jawad H, Ali NN, Lyon AR, Chen QZ, Harding SE, Boccaccini AR. Myocardial Tissue Engineering: a Review. Journal of Tissue Engineering and Regenerative Medicine 2007; 1: 327–342.

[27] Nelson DM, Mab Z, Fujimoto KL, Hashizume R, Wagner WR. Intra-Myocardial Biomaterial Injection Therapy in the Treatment of Heart Failure: Materials, Outcomes and Challenges. Acta Biomaterialia 2011; 7: 1-15.

[28] Chachques JC, Salanson-Lajos C, Lajos P, Shafy A, Alshamry A, Carpentier A. Cellular Cardiomyoplasty for Myocardial Regeneration. Asian Cardiovascular & Thoracic Annals 2005; 13: 287-296.

[29] Chen QZ, Harding SE, Ali NN, Lyon AR, Boccaccini AR. Biomaterials in Cardiac Tissue Engineering: Ten Years of Research Survey. Materials Science and Engineering 2008; 59: 1-37.

[30] Anversa P, Leri A, Kajstura J, Nadal-Ginard B. Myocyte Growth and Cardiac Repair. Journal of Molecular and Cellular Cardiology 2002; 34: 91-105.

[31] Bergmann O, Bhardwaj RD, Bernard S, Zdunek S, Barnabe-Heider F, Walsh S, Zupicich J, Alkass K, Buchholz BA, Druid H, Jovinge S, Frisén J. Evidence for Cardiomyocyte Renewal in Humans. Science 2009; 324(5923): 98-102.

[32] Wang F, Guan J. Cellular Cardiomyoplasty and Cardiac Tissue Engineering for Myocardial Therapy. Advanced Drug Delivery Reviews 2010; 62: 784–797.

[33] Chachques JC, Grandjean PA, Tommasi JJ, Perier P, Chauvaud S, Bourgeois I, Carpentier A. Dynamic Cardiomyoplasty: A New Approach to Assist Chronic Myocardial Failure. Life Support System 1987; 5(4): 323-7.

[34] Chachques JC. Development of Bioartificial Myocardium Using Stem Cells and Nanobiotechnology Templates. Cardiology Research and Practice 2011; 2011: 806795. doi:10.4061/2011/806795.

[35] Wu J, Zeng F, Weisel RD, Li RK. Stem Cells for Cardiac Regeneration by Cell Therapy and Myocardial Tissue Engineering. Advances in Biochemical Engineering/Biotechnology 2009; 114: 107-128. doi: 10.1007/10_2008_37.

[36] Pendyala L, Goodchild T, Gadesam RR, Chen J, Robinson K, Chronos N, Hou D. Cellular cardiomyoplasty and cardiac regeneration. Current Cardiology Reviews 2008; 4: 72-80.

[37] Leor J, Amsalem Y, Cohen S. Cells, scaffolds, and molecules for myocardial tissue engineering. Pharmacology and Therapeutics 2005; 105(2): 151-63.

[38] Zhou R, Acton PD, Ferrari VA. Imaging stem cells implanted in infarcted myocardium. Journal American college of cardiology 2006; 48(10): 2094-2106.

[39] Hofmann M, Wollert KC, Meyer GP, Menke A, Arseniev L, Hertenstein B, Ganser A, Knapp WH, Drexler H. Monitoring of Bone Marrow Cell Homing into the Infarcted Human Myocardium. Circulation 2005; 111: 2198-202.

[40] Teng CJ, Luo J, Chiu RC, Shum-Tim D. Massive Mechanical Loss of Microspheres with Direct Intramyocardial Injection in the Beating Heart: Implications for Cellular Cardiomyoplasty. Journal of Thoracic and Cardiovascular Surgery 2006; 132(3): 628-32. doi: 10.1016/j.jtcvs.2006.05.034.

[41] Schussler O, Chachques JC, Mesana TG, Suuronen EJ, Lecarpentier Y, Ruel M. 3-Dimensional structures to enhance cell therapy and engineer contractile tissue. Asian Cardiovascular & thoracic annals 2010; 18(2): 188-198.

[42] Zenovich AG, Davis BH, Taylor DA. Comparison of Intracardiac Cell Transplantation: Autologous Skeletal Myoblasts Versus Bone Marrow Cells. Handbook of Experimental Pharmacology 2007; 180: 117–165.

[43] Forte E, Chimenti I, Barile L, Gaetani R, Angelini F, Ionta V, Messina E, Giacomello A. Cardiac Cell Therapy: The Next (Re)Generation. Stem Cell Reviews and Reports 2011; 7(4): 1018-1030. doi:10.1007/s12015-011-9252-8.

[44] Qian H, Yang Y, Huang J, Dou K, Yang G. Cellular cardiomyoplasty by catheter-based infusion of stem cells in clinical settings. Transplant Immunology 2006; 16: 135-147.

[45] Laflamme MA, Chen KY, Naumova AV, Muskheli V, Fugate JA, Dupras SK, Reinecke H, Xu C, Hassanipour M, Police S, O'Sullivan C, Collins L, Chen Y, Minami E, Gill EA, Ueno S, Yuan C, Gold J, Murry CE. Cardiomyocytes derived from human embryonic stem cells in pro-survival factors enhance function of infarcted rat hearts. Nature Biotechnology 2007; 25(9): 1015-24. doi:10.1038/nbt1327.

[46] Ebelt H, Jungblut M, Zhang Y, Kubin T, Kostin S, Technau A, Oustanina S, Niebrügge S, Lechmann J, Werdan K, Braun T. Cellular cardiomyoplasty: improvement of left ventricular function correlates with the release of cardioactive cytokines. Stem cells 2007; 25(1): 236-244.

[47] Zimmet JM, Hare JM. Emerging role for bone marrow derived mesenchymal stem cells in myocardial regenerative therapy. Basic Research in Cardiology 2005; 100(6): 471-481. doi: 10.1007/s00395-005-0553-4.

[48] Madonna R, Geng YJ, De Caterina R. Adipose tissue-derived stem cells: characterization and potential for cardiovascular repair. Arteriosclerosis, Thrombosis and Vascular Biology 2009; 29(11): 1723-9.

[49] Heng BC, Haider HK, Sim EK, Cao T, Ng SC. Strategies for Directing the Differentiation of Stem Cells into the Cardiomyogenic Lineage in Vitro. Cardiovascular Research 2004; 62(1): 34–42.

[50] Vulliet PR, Greeley M, Halloran SM, MacDonald KA, Kittleson MD. Intra-Coronary
      Arterial Injection of Mesenchymal Stromal Cells and Microinfarction in Dogs. The
      Lancet 2004; 363(9411): 783-4.

[51] Meyer GP, Wollert KC, Lotz J, Steffens J, Lippolt P, Fichtner S, Hecker H, Schaefer A,
      Arseniev L, Hertenstein B, Ganser A, Drexler H. Intracoronary Bone Marrow Cell
      Transfer After Myocardial Infarction: Eighteen Months Follow-up Data from the
      Randomized, Controlled BOOST (BOne marrOw transfer to enhance ST-elevation in-
      farct regeneration) Trial. Circulation 2006; 113: 1287–94, doi: 10.1161/CIRCULATIO-
      NAHA.105.575118.

[52] Hahn JY, Cho HJ, Kang HJ, Kim TS, Kim MH, Chung JH, Bae JW, Oh BH, Park YB,
      Kim HS. Pre-treatment of Mesenchymal Stem Cells with a Combination of Growth
      Factors Enhances Gap Junction Formation, Cytoprotective Effect on Cardiomyocytes,
      and Therapeutic Efficacy for Myocardial Infarction. Journal of the American College
      of Cardiology 2008; 51(9): 933-43.

[53] Miyahara Y, Nagaya N, Kataoka M, Yanagawa B, Tanaka K, Hao H, Ishino K, Ishida
      H, Shimizu T, Kangawa K, Sano S, Okano T, Kitamura S, Mori H. Monolayered mes-
      enchymal stem cells repair scarred myocardium after myocardial infarction. Nature
      Medicine 2006; 12(4): 459-465.

[54] www.clinicaltrials.gov (accessed 13 November 2012).

[55] REgeneration of CArdiac Tissue Assisted by Bioactive Implants. funded by the Euro-
      pean Comission under the 7th FP, www.recatabi.com.

[56] Messina E, De Angelis L, Frati G, Morrone S, Chimenti S, Fiordaliso F, Salio M, Batta-
      glia M, Latronico MV, Coletta M, Vivarelli E, Frati L, Cossu G, Giacomello A. Isola-
      tion and Expansion of Adult Cardiac Stem Cells From Human and Murine Heart.
      Circulation Research 2004; 95: 911-921.

[57] Smith RR, Barile L, Cho HC, Leppo MK, Hare JM, Messina E, Giacomello A, Abra-
      ham MR, Marbán E. Regenerative potential of cardiosphere-derived cells expanded
      from percutaneous endomyocardial biopsy specimens. Circulation 2007; 115(7):
      896-908.

[58] Makkar RR, Smith RR, Cheng K, Malliaras K, Thomson LEJ, Berman D, Czer LSC,
      Marbán L, Mendizabal A, Johnston PV, Russell SD, Schuleri KH, Lardo AC, Gersten-
      blith G, Marbán E. Intracoronary cardiosphere-derived cells for heart regeneration
      after myocardial infarction (CADUCEUS): a prospective, randomised phase 1 trial.
      The Lancet 2012; 379: 895-904. doi: 10.1016/S0140- 6736(12)60195-0.

[59] Shafy A, Lavergne T, Latremouille C, Cortes-Morichetti M, Carpentier A, Chachques
      JC. Association of electrostimulation with cell transplantation in ischemic heart dis-
      ease. Journal of Thoracic and Cardiovascular Surgery 2009; 138(4): 994-1001.

[60] Cleland JG, Coletta AP, Abdellah AT, Nasirb M, Hobsonb N, Freemantlec N, Clarka
      AL. Clinical Trials Update from the American Heart Association 2006: OAT, SALT 1

and 2, MAGIC, ABCD, PABA-CHF, IMPROVECHF, and Percutaneous Mitral Annuloplasty. European Journal of Heart Failure 2007; 9: 92-7.

[61] Hirata Y, Sata M, Motomura N, Takanashi M, Suematsu Y, Ono M, Takamoto S. Human umbilical cord blood cells improve cardiac function after myocardial infarction. Biochemical and Biophysical Research Communications 2005; 327(2): 609-14. doi: 10.1016/j.bbrc.2004.12.044.

[62] Walther G, Gekas J, Bertrand OF. Amniotic Stem Cells for Cellular Cardiomyoplasty: Promises and Premises. Catheterization and Cardiovascular Interventions 2009; 73(7): 917–924.

[63] Yeh YC, Wei HJ, Lee WY, Yu CL, Chang Y, Hsu LW, Chung MF, Tsai MS, Hwang SM, Sung HW. Cellular Cardiomyoplasty with Human Amniotic Fluid Stem Cells: In Vitro and In Vivo Studies. Tissue Engineering Part A 2010; 16(6): 1925-36.

[64] Shimizu T, Yamato M, Kikuchi A, Okano T. Cell sheet engineering for myocardial tissue reconstruction. Biomaterials 2003; 24(13): 2309-2316.

[65] Alcon A, Cagavi Bozkulak E, Qyang Y. Regenerating functional heart tissue for myocardial repair. Cellular and Molecular Life Sciences 2012; 69(16): 2635-56. doi:10.1007/s00018-012-0942.

[66] Yeh YC, Lee WY, Yu CL, Hwang SM, Chung MF, Hsu LW, Chang Y, Lin WW, Tsai MS, Wei HJ, Sung HW. Cardiac repair with injectable cell sheet fragments of human amniotic fluid stem cells in an immune-suppressed rat model. Biomaterials 2010; 31(25): 6444-53.

[67] Furuta A, Miyoshi S, Itabashi Y, Shimizu T, Kira S, Hayakawa K, Nishiyama N, Tanimoto K, Hagiwara Y, Satoh T, Fukuda K, Okano T, Ogawa S. Pulsatile cardiac tissue grafts using a novel three-dimensional cell sheet manipulation technique functionally integrates with the host heart, in vivo. Circulation Research 2006; 98(5): 705–712.

[68] Williams C, Xie AW, Yamato M, Okano T, Wong JY. Stacking of aligned cell sheets for layer-by-layer control of complex tissue Structure. Biomaterials 2011; 32(24): 5625-32.

[69] Vunjak-Novakovic G, Lui KO, Tandon N, Chien KR. Bioengineering Heart Muscle: A Paradigm for Regenerative Medicine. Annual Reviewof Biomedical Engineering 2011; 13: 245–67. doi: 10.1146/annurev-bioeng-071910-124701.

[70] Haraguchi Y, Shimizu T, Yamato M, Kikuchi A, Okano T. Electrical coupling of cardiomyocyte sheets occurs rapidly via functional gap junction formation. Biomaterials 2006; 27(27): 4765–4774.

[71] Shimizu T, Sekine H, Yang J, Isoi Y, Yamato M, Kikuchi A, Kobayashi E, Okano T. Polysurgery of cell sheet grafts overcomes diffusion limits to produce thick, vascularized myocardial tissues. The Journal of the Federation of American Societies for Experimental Biology 2006; 20(6): 708–710.

[72] Lee WY, Wei HJ, Lin WW, Yeh YC, Hwang SM, Wang JJ, Tsai MS, Chang Y, Sung HW. Enhancement of cell retention and functional benefits in myocardial infarction using human amniotic-fluid stem-cell bodies enriched with endogenous ECM. Biomaterials 2011; 32(24): 5558-67.

[73] Ye Z, Zhou Y, Cai H, Tan W. Myocardial regeneration: Roles of stem cells and hydrogels. Advanced Drug Delivery Reviews 2011; 63(8): 688-97.

[74] Habib M, Shapira-Schweitzer K, Caspi O, Gepstein A, Arbel G, Aronson D, Seliktar D, Gepstein L. A combined cell therapy and in-situ tissue-engineering approach for myocardial repair. Biomaterials 2011; 32(30): 7514-23.

[75] Wall ST, Walker JC, Healy KE, Ratcliffe MB, Guccione JM. Theoretical impact of the injection of material into the myocardium: a finite element model simulation. Circulation 2006; 114(24): 2627-35.

[76] Shen X, Tanaka K, Takamori A. Coronary Arteries Angiogenesis in Ischemic Myocardium: Biocompatibility and Biodegradability of Various Hydrogels. Artificial Organs 2009; 33(10): 781-7. doi: 10.1111/j.1525-1594.2009.00815.x.

[77] Guo HD, Wang HJ, Tan YZ, Wu JH. Transplantation of marrow derived cardiac stem cells carried in fibrin improves cardiac function after myocardial infarction. Tissue Engineering Part A 2011; 17(1-2): 45-58.

[78] Christman KL, Vardanian AJ, Fang Q, Sievers RE, Fok HH, Lee RJ. Injectable fibrin scaffold improves cell transplant survival, reduces infarct expansion, and induces neovasculature formation in ischemic myocardium. Journal of the American College of Cardiology 2004; 44(3): 654-60.

[79] Barsotti MC, Felice F, Balbarini A, Di Stefano R. Fibrin as a scaffold for cardiac tissue Engineering. Biotechnology and Applied Biochemistry 2011; 58(5): 301-10. doi: 10.1002/bab.49.

[80] Christman KL, Fang Q, Yee MS, Johnson KR, Sievers RE, Lee RJ. Enhanced neovasculature formation in ischemic myocardium following delivery of pleiotrophin plasmid in a biopolymer. Biomaterials 2005; 26(10): 1139-44.

[81] Martens TP, Godier AF, Parks JJ, Wan LQ, Koeckert MS, Eng GM, Hudson BI, Sherman W, Vunjak-Novakovic G. Percutaneous cell delivery into the heart using hydrogels polymerizing in situ. Cell Transplantation 2009; 18(3): 297-304.

[82] Christman KL, Fok HH, Sievers RE, Fang Q, Lee RJ. Fibrin glue alone and skeletal myoblasts in a fibrin scaffold preserve cardiac function after myocardial infarction. Tissue Engineering 2004; 10 (3-4): 403-9.

[83] Ryu JH, Kim IK, Cho SW, Cho MC, Hwang KK, Piao H, Piao S, Lim SH, Hong YS, Choi CY, Yoo KJ, Kim BS. Implantation of bone marrow mononuclear cells using injectable fibrin matrix enhances neovascularization in infarcted myocardium. Biomaterials 2005; 26(3): 319–326.

[84] Chekanov V, Akhtar M, Tchekanov G, Dangas G, Shehzad MZ, Tio F, Adamian M, Colombo A, Roubin G, Leon MB, Moses JW, Kipshidze NN. Transplantation of autologous endothelial cells induces angiogenesis. Pacing and Clinical Electrophysiology 2003; 26(1 Pt 2): 496-9.

[85] Chenite A, Chaput C, Wang D, Combes C, Buschmann MD, Hoemann CD, Leroux JC, Atkinson BL, Binette F, Selmani A. Novel injectable neutral solutions of chitosan form biodegradable gels in situ. Biomaterials 2000; 21(21): 2155-61.

[86] Reis LA, Chiu LL, Liang Y, Hyunh K, Momen A, Radisic M. A peptide-modified chitosan–collagen hydrogel for cardiac cell culture and delivery. Acta Biomaterialia 2012; 8(3): 1022-36.

[87] Liu Z, Wang H, Wang Y, Lin Q, Yao A, Cao F, Li D, Zhou J, Duan C, Du Z, Wang Y, Wang C. The influence of chitosan hydrogel on stem cell engraftment, survival and homing in the ischemic myocardial microenvironment. Biomaterials 2012; 33(11): 3093-106.

[88] Binsalamah ZM, Paul A, Khan AA, Prakash S, Shum-Tim D. Intramyocardial sustained delivery of placental growth factor using nanoparticles as a vehicle for delivery in the rat infarct model. International Journal of Nanomedicine 2011; 6: 2667-78.

[89] Kofidis T, Lebl DR, Martinez EC, Hoyt G, Tanaka M, Robbins RC. Novel injectable bioartificial tissue facilitates targeted, less invasive, large-scale tissue restoration on the beating heart after myocardial injury. Circulation 2005; 112(9 Suppl): I173-7.

[90] Zhang P, Zhang H, Wang H, Wei Y, Hu S. Artificial matrix helps neonatal cardiomyocytes restore injured myocardium in rats. Artificial Organs 2006; 30(2): 86-93.

[91] Kofidis T, de Bruin JL, Hoyt G, Lebl DR, Tanaka M, Yamane T, Chang CP, Robbins RC. Injectable bioartificial myocardial tissue for large-scale intramural cell transfer and functional recovery of injured heart muscle. The Journal of Thoracic and Cardiovascular Surgery 2004; 128(4): 571-8.

[92] Shen D, Wang X, Zhang L, Zhao X, Li J, Cheng K, Zhang J. The amelioration of cardiac dysfunction after myocardial infarction by the injection of keratin biomaterials derived from human hair. Biomaterials 2011; 32(35): 9290-9.

[93] Landa N, Miller L, Feinberg MS, Holbova R, Shachar M, Freeman I, Cohen S, Leor J. Effect of injectable alginate implant on cardiac remodeling and function after recent and old infarcts in rat. Circulation 2008; 117(11): 1388-96.

[94] Ruvinov E, Leor J, Cohen S. The promotion of myocardial repair by the sequential delivery of IGF-1 and HGF from an injectable alginate biomaterial in a model of acute myocardial infarction. Biomaterials 2011; 32(2): 565-78.

[95] Rowley JA, Madlambayan G, Mooney DJ. Alginate hydrogels as synthetic extracellular matrix materials. Biomaterials 1999; 20(1): 45-53.

[96] Yu J, Gu Y, Du KT, Mihardja S, Sievers RE, Lee RJ. The effect of injected RGD modified alginate on angiogenesis and left ventricular function in a chronic rat infarct model. Biomaterials 2009; 30(5): 751-6.

[97] Tsur-Gang O, Ruvinov E, Landa N, Holbova R, Feinberg MS, Leor J, Cohen S. The effects of peptide-based modification of alginate on left ventricular remodeling and function after myocardial infarction. Biomaterials 2009; 30(2): 189-95.

[98] Mihardja SS, Sievers RE, Lee RJ. The effect of polypyrrole on arteriogenesis in an acute rat infarct model. Biomaterials 2008; 29(31): 4205-10.

[99] Gaffney J, Matou-Nasri S, Grau-Olivares M, Slevin M. Therapeutic applications of hyaluronan. Molecular BioSystems 2010; 6(3): 437–443. doi: 10.1039/b910552m.

[100] Yoon SJ, Fang YH, Lim CH, Kim BS, Son HS, Park Y, Sun K. Regeneration of ischemic heart using hyaluronic acid-based injectable hydrogel. Journal of Biomedical Materials Research Part B: Applied Biomaterials 2009; 91(1): 163-71.

[101] Cheng K, Blusztajn A, Shen D, Li TS, Sun B, Galang G, Zarembinski TI, Prestwich GD, Marbán E, Smith RR, Marbán L. Functional performance of human cardiosphere-derived cells delivered in an in situ polymerizable hyaluronan-gelatin hydrogel. Biomaterials 2012; 33(21): 5317-24.

[102] Duan Y, Liu Z, O'Neill J, Wan LQ, Freytes DO, Vunjak-Novakovic G. Hybrid gel composed of native heart matrix and collagen induces cardiac differentiation of human embryonic stem cells without supplemental growth factors. Journal of Cardiovascular Translational Research 2011; 4(5): 605-15.

[103] Dai W, Wold LE, Dow JS, Kloner RA. Thickening of the infarcted wall by collagen injection improves left ventricular function in rats: a novel approach to preserve cardiac function after myocardial infarction. Journal of the American College of Cardiology 2005; 46(4): 714-9.

[104] Huang NF, Yu J, Sievers R, Li S, Lee RJ. Injectable biopolymers enhance angiogenesis after myocardial infarction. Tissue Engineering 2005; 11(11-12): 1860-6.

[105] Thompson CA, Nasseri BA, Makower J, Houser S, McGarry M, Lamson T, Pomerantseva I, Chang JY, Gold HK, Vacanti JP, Oesterle SN. Percutaneous transvenous cellular cardiomyoplasty. A novel nonsurgical approach for myocardial cell transplantation. Journal of the American College of Cardiology 2003; 41(11): 1964-71.

[106] Dai W, Hale SL, Kay GL, Jyrala AJ, Kloner RA. Delivering stem cells to the heart in a collagen matrix reduces relocation of cells to other organs as assessed by nanoparticle technology. Regenerative Medicine 2009; 4(3): 387-95.

[107] Suuronen EJ, Veinot JP, Wong S, Kapila V, Price J, Griffith M, Mesana TG, Ruel M. Tissue-engineered injectable collagen-based matrices for improved cell delivery and vascularization of ischemic tissue using CD133+ progenitors expanded from the peripheral blood. Circulation 2006; 114(1 Suppl): I138-44.

[108] Zhang F, He C, Cao L, Feng W, Wang H, Mo X, Wang J. Fabrication of gelatin–hyaluronic acid hybrid scaffolds with tunable porous structures for soft tissue engineering. International Journal of Biological Macromolecules 2011; 48(3): 474-81.

[109] Shao ZQ, Takaji K, Katayama Y, Kunitomo R, Sakaguchi H, Lai ZF, Kawasuji M. Effects of intramyocardial administration of slow-release basic fibroblast growth factor on angiogenesis and ventricular remodeling in a rat infarct model. Circulation Journal 2006; 70(4): 471-7.

[110] Iwakura A, Fujita M, Kataoka K, Tambara K, Sakakibara Y, Komeda M, Tabata Y. Intramyocardial sustained delivery basic fibroblast growth factor improves angiogenesis and ventricular function in a rat infarct model. Heart Vessels 2003; 18: 93–9.

[111] Singelyn JM, DeQuach JA, Seif-Naraghi SB, Littlefield RB, Schup-Magoffin PJ, Christman KL. Naturally derived myocardial matrix as an injectable scaffold for cardiac tissue engineering. Biomaterials 2009; 30(29): 5409-16.

[112] Okada M, Payne TR, Oshima H, Momoi N, Tobita K, Huard J. Differential efficacy of gels derived from small intestinal submucosa as an injectable biomaterial for myocardial infarct repair. Biomaterials 2010; 31(30): 7678-83.

[113] Zhao ZQ, Puskas JD, Xu D, Wang NP, Mosunjac M, Guyton RA, Vinten-Johansen J, Matheny R. Improvement in cardiac function with small intestine extracellular matrix is associated with recruitment of C-kit cells, myofibroblasts, and macrophages after myocardial infarction. Journal of the American College of Cardiology 2010; 55(12): 1250-61.

[114] Jeong B, Kim SW, Bae YH. Thermosensitive sol-gel reversible hydrogels. Advanced Drug Delivery Reviews 2002; 54(1): 37-51.

[115] Fujimoto KL, Ma Z, Nelson DM, Hashizume R, Guan J, Tobita K, Wagner WR. Synthesis, characterization and therapeutic efficacy of a biodegradable, thermoresponsive hydrogel designed for application in chronic infarcted myocardium. Biomaterials 2009; 30(26): 4357-68.

[116] Li Z, Guo X, Matsushita S, Guan J. Differentiation of cardiosphere-derived cells into a mature cardiac lineage using biodegradable poly(N-isopropylacrylamide) hydrogels. Biomaterials 2011; 32(12): 3220-32.

[117] Wang T, Wu DQ, Jiang XJ, Zhang XZ, Li XY, Zhang JF, Zheng ZB, Zhuo R, Jiang H, Huang C. Novel thermosensitive hydrogel injection inhibits post-infarct ventricle remodelling. European Journal of Heart Failure 2009; 11(1): 14-9.

[118] Dobner S, Bezuidenhout D, Govender P, Zilla P, Davies N. Asynthetic nondegradable polyethylene glycol hydrogel retards adverse post-infarct left ventricular remodeling. Journal of Cardiac Failure 2009; 15(7): 629-36.

[119] Wang T, Jiang XJ, Tang QZ, Li XY, Lin T, Wu DQ, Zhang XZ, Okello E. Bone marrow stem cells implantation with a-cyclodextrin/MPEG– PCL–MPEG hydrogel improves cardiac function after myocardial infarction. Acta Biomaterialia 2009; 5(8): 2939-44.

[120] Wu J, Zeng F, Huang XP, Chung JC, Konecny F, Weisel RD, Li RK. Infarct stabilization and cardiac repair with a VEGF-conjugated, injectable Hydrogel. Biomaterials 2011; 32(2): 579-86.

[121] Kraehenbuehl TP, Ferreira LS, Hayward AM, Nahrendorf M, van der Vlies AJ, Vasile E, Weissleder R, Langer R, Hubbell JA. Human embryonic stem cell-derived microvascular grafts for cardiac tissue preservation after myocardial infarction. Biomaterials 2011; 32(4): 1102-9.

[122] Wang T, Jiang XJ, Lin T, Ren S, Li XY, Zhang XZ, Tang QZ. The inhibition of postinfarct ventricle remodeling without polycythaemia following local sustained intramyocardial delivery of erythropoietin within a supramolecular hydrogel. Biomaterials 2009; 30(25): 4161-7.

[123] Dvir T, Bauer M, Schroeder A, Tsui JH, Anderson DG, Langer R, Liao R, Kohane DS. Nanoparticles targeting the infarcted heart. Nano Letters 2011; 11(10): 4411-4. doi: 10.1021/nl2025882.

[124] Davis ME, Motion JP, Narmoneva DA, Takahashi T, Hakuno D, Kamm RD, Zhang S, Lee RT. Injectable self-assembling peptide nanofibers create intramyocardial microenvironments for endothelial cells.Circulation 2005; 111(4): 442-50.

[125] Tokunaga M, Liu ML, Nagai T, Iwanaga K, Matsuura K, Takahashi T, Kanda M, Kondo N, Wang P, Naito AT, Komuro I. Implantation of cardiac progenitor cells using self-assembling peptide improves cardiac function after myocardial infarction. Journal of Molecular and Cellular Cardiology 2010; 49(6): 972-83.

[126] Kim JH, Jung Y, Kim SH, Sun K, Choi J, Kim HC, Park Y, Kim SH. The enhancement of mature vessel formation and cardiac function in infarcted hearts using dual growth factor delivery with self-assembling peptides. Biomaterials 2011; 32(26): 6080-8.

[127] Davis ME, Hsieh PC, Takahashi T, Song Q, Zhang S, Kamm RD, Grodzinsky AJ, Anversa P, Lee RT. Local myocardial insulin-like growth factor 1 (IGF-1) delivery with biotinylated peptide nanofibers improves cell therapy for myocardial infarction. Proceedings of the National Academy of Sciences of the United States of America 2006; 103(21): 8155-60.

[128] Nerem RM. The challenge of imitating nature. In Lanza R, Langer R, Vacanti J.. Principles of tissue engineering. San Diego (Ca) USA: Academic press; 1997 p.9-15.

[129] Jawad H, Lyon AR, Harding SE, Ali NN, Boccaccini AR. Myocardial tissue engineering. British Medical Bulletin 2008; 87: 31-47.

[130] Engelmayr GC Jr, Cheng M, Bettinger CJ, Borenstein JT, Langer R, Freed LE. Accordion-like honeycombs for tissue engineering of cardiac anisotropy. Nature Materials 2008; 7: 1003–10.

[131] Bhana B, Iyer RK, Chen WL, Zhao R, Sider KL, Likhitpanichkul M, Simmons CA, Radisic M. Influence of substrate stiffness on the phenotype of heart cells. Biotechnology and Bioengineering 2010; 105(6): 1148-60.

[132] Marsano A, Maidhof R, Wan LQ, Wang Y, Gao J, Tandon N, Vunjak-Novakovic G. Scaffold stiffness affects the contractile function of three-dimensional engineered cardiac constructs. Biotechnology Progress 2010; 26(5): 1382-90.

[133] Young JL, Engler AJ. Hydrogels with time-dependent material properties enhance cardiomyocyte differentiation in vitro. Biomaterials 2011; 32(4): 1002-9.

[134] Carrier RL, Rupnick M, Langer R, Schoen FJ, Freed LE, Vunjak-Novakovic G. Perfusion Improves Tissue Architecture of Engineered Cardiac Muscle. Tissue Engineering 2002; 8(2): 175-88.

[135] Radisic M, Malda J, Epping E, Geng W, Langer R, Vunjak-Novakovic G. Oxygen gradients correlate with cell density and cell viability in engineered cardiac tissue. Biotechnology and Bioengineering 2006; 93(2): 332-43.

[136] Radisic M, Park H, Chen F, Salazar-Lazzaro JE, Wang Y, Dennis R, Langer R, Freed LE, Vunjak-Novakovic G. Biomimetic approach to cardiac tissue engineering: oxygen carriers and channeled scaffolds. Tissue Engineering 2006; 12(8): 2077-91.

[137] Perets A, Baruch Y, Weisbuch F, Shoshany G, Neufeld G, Cohen S. Enhancing the vascularization of three-dimensional porous alginate scaffolds by incorporating controlled release basic fibroblast growth factor microspheres. Journal of Biomedical Materials Research Part A 2003; 65(4): 489-97.

[138] Miyagi Y, Chiu LL, Cimini M, Weisel RD, Radisic M, Li RK. Biodegradable collagen patch with covalently immobilized VEGF for myocardial repair. Biomaterials 2011; 32(5): 1280-90.

[139] Chiu LL, Radisic M. Controlled release of thymosin β4 using collagen–chitosan composite hydrogels promotes epicardial cell migration and angiogenesis. Journal of Controlled Release 2011; 155(3): 376-85. doi: 10.1016/j.jconrel.2011.05.026.

[140] Vantler M, Karikkineth BC, Naito H, Tiburcy M, Didié M, Nose M, Rosenkranz S, Zimmermann WH. PDGF-BB protects cardiomyocytes from apoptosis and improves contractile function of engineered heart tissue. Journal of Molecular and Cellular Cardiology 2010; 48(6): 1316-23.

[141] Davis ME, Hsieh PC, Grodzinsky AJ, Lee RT. Custom design of the cardiac microenvironment with biomaterials. Circulation Research 2005; 97(1): 8-15.

[142] Kaully T, Kaufman-Francis K, Lesman A, Levenberg S. Vascularization--the conduit to viable engineered tissues. Tissue Engineering Part B Reviews 2009; 15(2): 159-69.

[143] Bar A, Haverich A, Hilfiker A. Cardiac tissue engineering: "Reconstructing the motor of life". Scandinavian Journal of surgery 2007; 96 (2): 154-8.

[144] Narmoneva DA, Vukmirovic R, DavisME, Kamm RD, Lee RT. Endothelial cells promote cardiacmyocyte survival and spatial reorganization: implications for cardiac regeneration. Circulation 2004; 110(8): 962-8.

[145] Dvir T, Kedem A, Ruvinov E, Levy O, Freeman I, Landa N, Holbova R, Feinberg MS, Dror S, Etzion Y, Leor J, Cohen S. Prevascularization of cardiac patch on the omentum improves its therapeutic outcome. Proceedings of the National Academy of Sciences from the United States of America 2009; 106 (35): 14990-5.

[146] Bursac N, Papadaki M, White JA, Eisenberg SR, Vunjak-Novakovic G, Freed LE. Cultivation in rotating bioreactors promotes maintenance of cardiac myocyte electrophysiology and molecular properties. Tissue Engineering 2003; 9(6): 1243-53.

[147] Radisic M, Yang L, Boublik J, Cohen RJ, Langer R, Freed LE, Vunjak-Novakovic G. Medium perfusion enables engineering of compact and contractile cardiac tissue. American Journal of Physiology Heart and Circulatory Physiology 2004; 286(2): H507-16.

[148] Radisic M, Marsano A, Maidhof R, Wang Y, Vunjak-Novakovic G. Cardiac tissue engineering using perfusion bioreactor systems. Nature Protocols 2008; 3(4): 719-38.

[149] Maidhof R, Marsano A, Lee EJ, Vunjak-Novakovic G. Perfusion Seeding of Channeled Elastomeric Scaffolds with Myocytes and Endothelial Cells for Cardiac Tissue Engineering. Biotechnology Progress 2010; 26(2): 565-72.

[150] Brown MA, Iyer RK, Radisic M. Pulsatile perfusion bioreactor for cardiac tissue engineering. Biotechnology Progress 2008; 24(4): 907-20.

[151] Cheng M, Moretti M, Engelmayr GC, Freed LE. Insulin-like Growth Factor-I and Slow, Bi-directional Perfusion Enhance the Formation of Tissue-Engineered Cardiac Grafts. Tissue Engineering Part A 2009; 15(3): 645-53.

[152] Li D, Xia Y. Electrospinning of nanofibers: reinventing the wheel? Advanced Materials 2004; 16(14): 1151–1170. doi: 10.1002/adma.200400719.

[153] Orlova Y, Magome N, Liu L, Chen Y, Agladze K. Electrospun nanofibers as a tool for architecture control in engineered cardiac tissue. Biomaterials 2011; 32(24): 5615-24.

[154] Blan NR, Birla RK. Design and fabrication of heart muscle using scaffold-based tissue engineering. Journal of Biomedical Materials Research Part A 2008; 86(1): 195-208.

[155] Madihally SV, Matthew HW. Porous chitosan scaffolds for tissue engineering. Biomaterials 1999; 20(12): 1133-42.

[156] Cimetta E, Pizzato S, Bollini S, Serena E, De Coppi P, Elvassore N. Production of arrays of cardiac and skeletal muscle myofibers by micropatterning techniques on a soft substrate. Biomedical Microdevices 2009; 11(2): 389-400.

[157] Chiang CK, Chowdhury MF, Iyer RK, Stanford WL, Radisic M. Engineering surfaces for site-specific vascular differentiation of mouse embryonic stem cells. Acta Biomaterialia 2010; 6(6): 1904-16.

[158] Park H, Radisic M, Lim JO, Chang BH, Vunjak-Novakovic G. A novel composite scaffold for cardiac tissue engineering. In Vitro Cellular and Developmental Biology Animal 2005; 41(7): 188-96.

[159] Eschenhagen T, Fink C, Remmers U, Scholz H, Wattchow J, Weil J, Zimmermann W, Dohmen HH, Schäfer H, Bishopric N, Wakatsuki T, Elson EL. Three-dimensional reconstitution of embryonic cardiomyocytes in a collagen matrix: a new heart muscle model system. The Journal of the Federation of American Societies for Experimental Biology 1997; 11(8): 683-94.

[160] Callegari A, Bollini S, Iop L, Chiavegato A, Torregrossa G, Pozzobon M, Gerosa G, De Coppi P, Elvassore N, Sartore S. Neovascularization induced by porous collagen scaffold implanted on intact and cryoinjured rat hearts. Biomaterials 2007; 28(36): 5449-61.

[161] Xiang Z, Liao R, Kelly MS, Spector M. Collagen-GAG scaffolds grafted onto myocardial infarcts in a rat model: a delivery vehicle for mesenchymal stem cells. Tissue Engineering 2006; 12(9): 2467-78.

[162] Simpson DL, Dudley SC Jr. Modulation of human mesenchymal stem cell function in a three-dimensional matrix promotes attenuation of adverse remodelling after myocardial infarction. Journal of Tissue Engineering and Regenerative Medicine 2011 Nov 18. doi: 10.1002/term.511.

[163] Chachques JC, Trainini JC, Lago N, Masoli OH, Barisani JL, Cortes-Morichetti M, Schussler O, Carpentier A. Myocardial assistance by grafting a new bioartificial upgraded myocardium (MAGNUM clinical trial): one year follow-up. Cell Transplantation 2007; 16(9): 927-34.

[164] Chimenti I, Rizzitelli G, Gaetani R, Angelini F, Ionta V, Forte E, Frati G, Schussler O, Barbetta A, Messina E, Dentini M, Giacomello A. Human cardiosphere-seeded gelatin and collagen scaffolds as cardiogenic engineered bioconstructs. Biomaterials 2011; 32(35): 9271-81.

[165] Holladay CA, Duffy AM, Chen X, Sefton MV, O'Brien TD, Pandit AS. Recovery of cardiac function mediated by MSC and interleukin-10 plasmid functionalised scaffold. Biomaterials 2012; 33(5): 1303-14.

[166] Akhyari P, Kamiya H, Haverich A, Karck M, Lichtenberg A. Myocardial tissue engi-
       neering: the extracellular matrix. Journal of Cardio-thoracic Surgery 2008; 34:
       229-241.

[167] Sakai T, Li RK, Weisel RD, Mickle DA, Kim ET, Jia ZQ, Yau TM. The fate of a tissue-
       engineered cardiac graft in the right ventricular outflow tract of the rat. Journal of
       Thoracic and Cardiovascular Surgery 2001; 121(5): 932-42.

[168] Zhang G, Nakamura Y, Wang X, Hu Q, Suggs LJ, Zhang J. Controlled release of stro-
       mal cell-derived factor-1 alpha in situ increases c-kit+ cell homing to the infarcted
       heart. Tissue Engineering 2007; 13(8): 2063-71.

[169] Leor J, Aboulafia-Etzion S, Dar A, Shapiro L, Barbash IM, Battler A, Granot Y, Cohen
       S. Bioengineered cardiac grafts: A new approach to repair the infarcted myocardi-
       um? Circulation 2000; 102(19 Suppl 3): III56-61.

[170] Dar A, Shachar M, Leor J, Cohen S. Optimization of cardiac cell seeding and distribu-
       tion in 3D porous alginate scaffolds. Biotechnology and Bioengineering 2002; 80(3):
       305-12.

[171] Shachar M, Tsur-Gang O, Dvir T, Leor J, Cohen S. The effect of immobilized RGD
       peptide in alginate scaffolds on cardiac tissue engineering. Acta Biomaterialia 2011;
       7(1): 152-62.

[172] Sapir Y, Kryukov O, Cohen S. Integration of multiple cell-matrix interactions into al-
       ginate scaffolds for promoting cardiac tissue regeneration. Biomaterials 2011; 32(7):
       1838-47.

[173] Le Visage C, Gournay O, Benguirat N, Hamidi S, Chaussumier L, Mougenot N, Flan-
       ders JA, Isnard R, Michel JB, Hatem S, Letourneur D, Norol F. Mesenchymal stem
       cell delivery into rat infarcted myocardium using a porous polysaccharide-based
       scaffold: a quantitative comparison with endocardial injection. Tissue Engineering
       Part A 2012; 18(1-2): 35-44.

[174] Cao Y, Wang B. Biodegradation of Silk Biomaterials. International Journal of Molecu-
       lar Sciences 2009; 10(4): 1514-1524.

[175] Yang MC, Wang SS, Chou NK, Chi NH, Huang YY, Chang YL, Shieh MJ, Chung TW.
       The cardiomyogenic differentiation of rat mesenchymal stem cells on silk fibroin–
       polysaccharide cardiac patches in vitro. Biomaterials 2009; 30(22): 3757-65.

[176] Patra C, Talukdar S, Novoyatleva T, Velagala SR, Mühlfeld C, Kundu B, Kundu SC,
       Engel FB. Silk protein fibroin for cardiac tissue engineering. Biomaterials 2012; 33(9):
       2673-80.

[177] Robinson KA, Li J, Mathison M, Redkar A, Cui J, Chronos NA, Matheny RG, Badylak
       SF. Extracellular matrix scaffold for cardiac repair. Circulation 2005; 112(9 Suppl):
       I135-43.

[178] Godier-Furnémont AF, Martens TP, Koeckert MS, Wan L, Parks J, Arai K, Zhang G, Hudson B, Homma S, Vunjak-Novakovic G. Composite scaffold provides a cell delivery platform for cardiovascular repair. Proceedings of the National Academy of Sciences of the United States of America 2011; 108(19): 7974-9.

[179] Wei HJ, Chen CH, Lee WY, Chiu I, Hwang SM, Lin WW, Huang CC, Yeh YC, Chang Y, Sung HW. Bioengineered cardiac patch constructed from multilayered mesenchymal stem cells for myocardial repair. Biomaterials 2008; 29(26): 3547-56.

[180] Ott HC, Matthiesen TS, Goh SK, Black LD, Kren SM, Netoff TI, Taylor DA. Perfusion-decellularized matrix: using nature's platform to engineer a bioartificial heart. Nature Medicine 2008; 14(2): 213-221.

[181] Giraud MN, Armbruster C, Carrel T, Tevaearai HT. Current state of the art in myocardial tissue engineering. Tissue Engineering 2007; 13(8): 1825-36.

[182] Huang CC, Wei HJ, Yeh YC, Wang JJ, Lin WW, Lee TY, Hwang SM, Choi SW, Xia Y, Chang Y, Sung HW. Injectable PLGA porous beads cellularized by hAFSCs for cellular cardiomyoplasty. Biomaterials 2012; 33(16): 4069-77.

[183] McDevitt TC, Angello JC, Whitney ML, Reinecke H, Hauschka SD, Murry CE, Stayton PS. In vitro generation of differentiated cardiac myofibers on micropatterned laminin surfaces. Journal of Biomedical Materials Research 2002; 60(3): 472-9.

[184] Stout DA, Basu B, Webster TJ. Poly(lactic–co-glycolic acid): Carbon nanofiber composites for myocardial tissue engineering applications. Acta Biomaterialia 2011; 7(8): 3101-12. doi:10.1016/j.actbio.2011.04.028 4.

[185] Caspi O, Lesman A, Basevitch Y, Gepstein A, Arbel G, Habib IH, Gepstein L, Levenberg S. Tissue engineering of vascularized cardiac muscle from human embryonic stem cells. Circulation Research 2007; 100(2): 263-72.

[186] Ishii O, Shin M, Sueda T, Vacanti JP. In vitro tissue engineering of a cardiac graft using a degradable scaffold with an extracellular matrix–like topography. Journal of Thoracic and Cardiovascular Surgery 2005; 130(5): 1358-63.

[187] Piao H, Kwon JS, Piao S, Sohn JH, Lee YS, Bae JW, Hwang KK, Kim DW, Jeon O, Kim BS, Park YB, Cho MC. Effects of cardiac patches engineered with bone marrow-derived mononuclear cells and PGCL scaffolds in a rat myocardial infarction model. Biomaterials 2007; 28(4): 641-9.

[188] Gorna K, Gogolewski S. Biodegradable polyurethanes for implants. II. In vitro degradation and calcification of materials from poly(epsilon-caprolactone)-poly(ethylene oxide) diols and various chain extenders. Journal of Biomedical Materials Research 2002; 60(4): 592-606.

[189] Zhang JY, Beckman EJ, Piesco NP, Agarwal S. A new peptide-based urethane polymer: synthesis, biodegradation, and potential to support cell growth in vitro. Biomaterials 2000; 21(12): 1247-1258.

[190] Rockwood DN, Akins RE Jr, Parrag IC, Woodhouse KA, Rabolt JF. Culture on elec-trospun polyurethane scaffolds decreases atrial natriuretic peptide expression by car-diomyocytes in vitro. Biomaterials 2008; 29(36): 4783-91. doi:10.1016/j.biomaterials. 2008.08.034.

[191] Guan J, Fujimoto KL, Sacks MS, Wagner WR. Preparation and characterization of highly porous, biodegradable polyurethane scaffolds for soft tissue applications. Bio-materials 2005; 26(18): 3961-3971. doi:10.1016/j.biomaterials.2004.10.018.

[192] Fujimoto KL, Tobita K, Merryman WD, Guan J, Momoi N, Stolz DB, Sacks MS, Keller BB, Wagner WR. An elastic, biodegradable cardiac patch induces contractile smooth muscle and improves cardiac remodeling and function in subacute myocardial in-farction. Journal of the American College of Cardiology 2007; 49(23): 2292-300. doi: 10.1016/j.jacc.2007.02.050.

[193] Siepe M, Giraud MN, Liljensten E, Nydegger U, Menasche P, Carrel T, Tevaearai HT. Construction of skeletal myoblast-based polyurethane scaffolds for myocardial re-pair. Artificial Organs 2007; 31(6): 425-33.

[194] Chen QZ, Bismarck A, Hansen U, Junaid S, Tran MQ, Harding SE, Ali NN, Boccacci-ni AR. Characterisation of a soft elastomer poly(glycerol sebacate) designed to match the mechanical properties of myocardial tissue. Biomaterials 2008; 29(1): 47-57.

[195] Jean A, Engelmayr GC Jr. Finite element analysis of an accordion-like honeycomb scaffold for cardiac tissue engineering. Journal of Biomechanics 2010; 43(15): 3035-43.

[196] Ravichandran R, Venugopal JR, Sundarrajan S, Mukherjee S, Ramakrishna S. Poly(glycerol sebacate)/gelatin core/shell fibrous structure for regeneration of myo-cardial infarction. Tissue Engineering Part A 2011; 17(9-10): 1363-73. doi: 10.1089/ ten.tea.2010.0441.

[197] Ifkovits JL, Devlin JJ, Eng G, Martens TP, Vunjak-Novakovic G, Burdick JA. Biode-gradable fibrous scaffolds with tunable properties formed from photo-cross-linkable poly(glycerol sebacate). ACS Applied Materials and Interfaces 2009; 1(9): 1878-86.

[198] Madden LR, Mortisen DJ, Sussman EM, Dupras SK, Fugate JA, Cuy JL, Hauch KD, Laflamme MA, Murry CE, Ratner BD. Proangiogenic scaffolds as functional tem-plates for cardiac tissue engineering. Proceedings of the National Academy of Scien-ces of the United States of America 2010; 107(34): 15211-6. doi: 10.1073/pnas. 1006442107.

[199] Arnal-Pastor M, Vallés-Lluch A, Keicher M, Pradas MM. Coating typologies and con-strained swelling of hyaluronic acid gels within scaffold pores. Journal of Colloid and Interface Science 2011; 361(1): 361-9.

[200] Sauer H, Rahimi G, Hescheler J, Wartenberg M. Effects of electrical fields on cardio-myocyte differentiation of embryonic stem cells. Journal of Cellular Biochemistry 1999; 75(4): 710–723.

[201] Haneef K, Lila N, Benadda S, Legrand F, Carpentier A, Chachques JC. Development of bioartificial myocardium by electrostimulation of 3D collagen scaffolds seeded with stem cells. Heart International 2012; 7(2): e14.

[202] Radisic M, Park H, Shing H, Consi T, Schoen FJ, Langer R, Freed LE, Vunjak-Novakovic G. Functional assembly of engineered myocardium by electrical stimulation of cardiac myocytes cultured on scaffolds. Proceedings of the National Academy of Sciences of the United States of America 2004; 101(52): 18129-34.

[203] Serena E, Figallo E, Tandon N, Cannizzaro C, Gerecht S, Elvassore N, Vunjak-Novakovic G. Electrical stimulation of human embryonic stem cells: Cardiac differentiation and the generation of reactive oxygen species. Experimental Cell Research 2009; 315(20): 3611-9.

[204] Tandon N, Marsanno A, Maidhof R, Wan L. Park H, Vunjak-Novakovic G. Optimization of electrical stimulation parameters for cardiac tissue engineering. Journal of Tissue Engineering and Regenerative Medicine 2011; 5: e115–e125.

[205] Tandon N, Marsano A, Maidhof R, Numata K, Montouri-Sorrentino C, Cannizzaro C, Voldmand J, Vunjak-Novakovic G. Surface-patterned electrode bioreactor for electrical stimulation. Lab on a Chip 2010; 10: 692–700.

[206] Dvir T, Timko BP, Brigham MD, Naik SR, Karajanagi SS, Levy O, Jin H, Parker KK, Langer R, Kohane DS. Nanowired three-dimensional cardiac patches. Nature Nanotechnology 2011; 6(11): 720-5. doi:10.1038/nnano.2011.160.

[207] You J-O, Rafat M, Ye GJC Auguste,DT. Nanoengineering the heart: conductive scaffolds enhance connexin 43 expression. Nano Letters 2011; 11(9): 3643–3648.

[208] Fink C, Ergün S, Kralisch D, Remmers U, Weil J, Eschenhagen T. Chronic stretch of engineered heart tissue induces hypertrophy and functional improvement. Federation of American Societies for Experimental Biology Journal 2000; 14(5): 669-79.

[209] Zimmermann WH, Schneiderbanger K, Schubert P, Didié M, Münzel M, Heubach F,Kostin S, Neuhuber WL, Eschenhagen T. Tissue engineering of a differentiated cardiac muscle construct. Circulation Research 2002; 90: 223-230.

[210] Guan J, Wang F, Li Z, Chen J, Guo X, Liao J, Moldovan NI. The stimulation of the cardiac differentiation of mesenchymal stem cells in tissue constructs that mimic myocardium structure and biomechanics. Biomaterials 2011; 32(24): 5568-80.

[211] Zhang T, Wan LQ, Xiong Z, Marsano A, Maidhof R, Park M, Yan Y, Vunjak-Novakovic G. Channelled scaffolds for engineering myocardium with mechanical stimulation. Journal of Tissue Engineering and Regenerative Medicine 2011. doi: 10.1002/term.481.

[212] Akhyari P, Fedak PW, Weisel RD, Lee TY, Verma S, Mickle DA, Li RK. Mechanical stretch regimen enhances the formation of bioengineered autologous cardiac muscle grafts. Circulation 2002; 106(12 Suppl 1): I137-42.

[213] Chachques JC, Jegaden O, Mesana T, Glock Y, Grandjean PA, Carpentier AF, et al. Cardiac bioassist: results of the French multicenter cardiomyoplasty study. Asian Cardiovascular and Thoracic Annals 2009; 17: 573-80.

[214] Kwon MH, Cevasco M, Schmitto JD, Chen FY. Ventricular restraint therapy for heart failure: A review, summary of state of the art, and future directions. Journal of Thoracic and Cardiovascular Surgery 2012; 144(4): 771-777.

[215] Liao SY, Siu CW, Liu Y, Zhang Y, Chan WS, Wu EX, Wu Y, Nicholls JM, Li RA, Benser ME, Rosenberg SP, Park E, Lau CP, Tse HF. Attenuation of left ventricular adverse remodeling with epicardial patching after myocardial infarction. Journal of Cardiac Failure 2010; 16 (7): 590-8.

[216] Enomoto Y, Gorman JH 3rd, Moainie SL, Jackson BM, Parish LM, Plappert T, Zeeshan A, St John-Sutton MG, Gorman RC. Early ventricular restraint after myocardial infarction: extent of the wrap determines the outcome of remodeling. Annals of Thoracic Surgery 2005; 79(3): 881-7.

[217] Klodell CT, Aranda JM, McGiffin DC, Rayburn BK, Sun B, Abraham WT, Pae WE, Boehmer JP, Klein H, Huth C. Worldwide surgical experience with the Paracor HeartNet cardiac restraint device. The Journal of Thoracic and Cardiovascular Surgery 2008; 135(1): 188–195.

[218] Costanzo MR, Ivanhoe RJ, Kao A, Anand IS, Bank A, Boehmer J, Demarco T, Hergert CM, Holcomb RG, Maybaum S, Sun B, Vassiliades TA Jr, Rayburn BK, Abraham WT. Prospective evaluation of elastic restraint to lessen the effects of heart failure (PEERLESS-HF) trial. Journal of Cardiac Failure 2012; 18(6): 446-58. doi: 10.1016/j.cardfail.2012.04.004.

[219] Dixon JA, Goodman AM, Gaillard WF 2nd, Rivers WT, McKinney RA, Mukherjee R, Baker NL, Ikonomidis JS, Spinale FG. Hemodynamics and myocardial blood flow patterns after placement of a cardiac passive restraint device in a model of dilated cardiomyopathy. Journal of Thoracic and Cardiovascular Surgery 2011; 142: 1038-45.

[220] Pilla JJ, Blom AS, Brockman DJ, Ferrari VA, Yuan Q, Acker MA. Passive ventricular constraint to improve left ventricular function and mechanics in an ovine model of heart failure secondary to acute myocardial infarction. Journal of Thoracic and Cardiovascular Surgery 2003; 126(5): 1467-76.

[221] Mann DL, Kubo SH, Sabbah HN, Starling RC, Jessup M, Oh JK, Acker MA. Beneficial effects of the CorCap cardiac support device: five-year results from the Acorn Trial. Journal of Thoracic and Cardiovascular Surgery 2012; 143(5): 1036-42.

[222] Olsson A, Bredin F, Franco-Cereceda A. Echocardiographic findings using tissue velocity imaging following passive containment surgery with the Acorn CorCap cardiac support device. European Journal of Cardio-Thoracic Surgery 2005; 28: 448-53.

[223] Shafy A, Fink T, Zachar V, Lilaa N, Carpentier A, Chachques JC. Development of cardiac support bioprostheses for ventricular restoration and myocardial regeneration. European Journal of Cardio-Thoracic Surgery 2012; 0: 1–9. doi:10.1093/ejcts/ezs480.

Chapter 2

The Evolution of Three-Dimensional Cell Cultures Towards Unimpeded Regenerative Medicine and Tissue Engineering

Aleksandar Evangelatov and Roumen Pankov

Additional information is available at the end of the chapter

1. Introduction

The idea that cellular survival and growth could be maintained outside the body was recognized as possible almost hundred years ago when the German zoologist Wilhelm Roux described a successful experiment where he cultured chick neural crest in warm saline for a few days [1]. Nobel Prize winner Alexis Carrel performed numerous experiments clearly showing that tissue explants, including connective tissue and heart tissue, could be cultured in vitro preserving their characteristics for prolonged periods of time [2] supporting the notion that entire organs could be cultured in vitro. A defined synthetic mixture of amino acids, salts, carbohydrates, vitamins and serum was shown to support cells in vitro[3], thus unifying a major variable in cell culturing experiments and providing a possibility for rapid development of this novel method. Since the establishment of the first cell line by Gey et al.[4] in 1951 cell culturing has become one of the most widely used methods with exceptional contribution to the advances in almost all fields of contemporary biology – cell biology, genetics, cell biochemistry, physiology etc. Significant progress in the field made possible numerous achievements that were believed to be the foundations of personalized medicine. Among these is the isolation of the first line of murine stem cells [5, 6] in 1981, followed by establishment of the first human embryonic stem cell lines by Thompson [7].

Current knowledge of cellular behavior is mainly acquired by studies concerning homogenous populations of cells cultured as monolayers. This simplified approach towards understanding the essence of the mechanisms, underlying the processes determining life and death of a cell has undoubtedly provided scientists with enormous amount of knowledge. However, recent advances in the field of three-dimensional cell cultures have revealed a lot of imperfections in this limiting approach. Growing fibroblasts on flat, rigid surface of the Petri dish or flask results in major differences in adhesion formation and maturation, proliferation, cell signaling, migration and cytoskeletal function, compared to the three-dimensional environment [8-12]. Even changes in stiffness of the two-dimensional (2D) substrate have shown significant difference in fibroblasts response to the environment [13, 14]. Being cultured on 2D surfaces, these non-polar cells are forced to adapt to polar setting, thus significantly changing their response to the environment. One could argue that this culturing method would be ideal for epithelial cells, allowing them to form distinct apical and basal layers. Nevertheless growth in 3D environment allows normal polarization and differentiation of epithelial cells [15] and is a prerequisite for the formation of duct-like structures in vitro [16]. Thereby the emerging differences between conventional, monolayer cell cultures and in vivo cellular behavior led to the increasing number of scientists aiming to provide in vivo-relevant results.

The idea of cell culturing in 3D environment is not a novel one though [17], but until recently the importance of the cell environment – its dimensionality, stiffness, elasticity, composition and remodeling during tissue morphogenesis and disease, remained neglected. Number of studies have shown that knockdown of extracellular matrix (ECM) components like fibronectin, collagen, laminin, aggrecan, etc. lead to lethal phenotypes or severe pathologies during embryonic or post-natal development [18-24]. Furthermore, recent discoveries like the importance of Cdc42 for the appropriate acquisition of apical and basal polarity during morphogenesis or cell specification during tubulogenesis wouldn't have been possible without the use of 3D model systems [25, 26]. Thus the concept of the importance of the surrounding settings emerged and an entirely new scientific direction evolved, focusing on the role of the extracellular matrix and its importance in cell biology.

In the living organism cells are usually embedded in a complex three-dimensional extracellular matrix that is dynamic in its structure[27] and rarely do have the opportunity to attach to planar, rigid substrates. Reciprocal interactions between cells and the ECM facilitate signaling to and from cells and lead to continuous reorganization of the environment [10]. Investigation of the dynamics of the ECM, its structure in different tissues and cellular response to changes in the mechanical properties of the extracellular matrices have shown that cells are not only able to feel and respond to the environment, but also to cause changes to the environment's mechanical properties [14]. These interactions deliver further signals responsible for cell growth and differentiation, survival, migration and reorganization of the resident tissue [28]. In addition when one thinks of cells in the third dimension it has to be considered that cells are not just randomly incorporated in the ECM but form complex 3D structures, characteristic of the specific tissue or organ [29].

The recognition of the importance of dimensionality of cellular environment encouraged the creation of a variety of three-dimensional culturing systems. Essentially they could be divided into two groups – three-dimensional systems made of artificial materials, mimicking the natural components of the matrix and three-dimensional culturing systems based on natural ECM components, or cell-synthesized ECM. This article's focus will be mainly on the later 3D culturing models.

2. Artificially fabricated 3D scaffolds

Design of artificial 3D environments for cells aims at creating an environment that would mimic the physical properties of the natural extracellular matrix along with the signaling cues it provides for cell development. Such scaffolds should be non-toxic, preferably biodegradable in time and must allow cell attachment and migration as well as diffusion of vital nutrients [30]. Cells should be able to proliferate and differentiate, and subsequently to synthesize and organize their own ECM. In time, eventually, the naturally synthesized and organized extracellular matrix should substitute the artificial scaffold. All those prerequisites mean that the surface should be suitable for cell attachment, have the adequate chemical and mechanical properties to support adhesion, proliferation and differentiation. To our knowledge there are currently several reported methods for fabricating appropriate artificial scaffolds:

- The technique of controlled rate freezing and lypohilization [31] produces suitable extracellular matrices, in spite of the relatively uneven pore sizes. Another drawback of this method is that the produced artificial matrix does not have fibrillar structure which is common for the natural ECM.

- Phase separation of nanofibers [32] yields fibrous matrices, but also produces pores with uneven sizes.

- Formation of porous scaffolds [33]. This method allows the formation of matrices with similar pore sizes, but is limited by the matrix thickness

- Computer-assisted design and manufacturing (CAD/CAM) technologies [34] allow the formation of geometrically complex structures, with precise control over pore sizes, variety of material choices, layering, etc. with the use of some biological materials. A drawback of these technologies is the lack of ability to produce fibrous structures in the nanoscale.

- Nanofiber self assembly of thinner fibrils [35] is a relatively expensive method, but allows the production of thinner than 10nm filaments that subsequently form thicker fibers, organizing structures, similar to the natural extracellular matrix.

- The electrospinning technology [36] is used to produce matrices of fibers in the micro- and nanoscale by employment of numerous polymers including also natural polymers. Even though this technique allows for much more precise tailoring of the biological and mechanical properties of the resulting matrices, it is still limited by the achieved small pore sizes thus limiting cellular migration within the matrix.

All these methods find application in medicinal practice and tissue engineering, but there are still many questions to be answered regarding their safety with long term usage, biodegradability, their influence on cellular signaling, proliferation and differentiation, etc. that are beyond the scope of this review.

3. 3D culturing systems based on natural components of the ECM

Gels present the easiest, most affordable and quickest way to provide cells with a three-dimensional environment that can be further manipulated by variety of methods in order to modulate their properties. Different types of gels have been utilized during the past few decades with collagen, fibrin, hyaluronan and basement membrane extract (BME) gels being the most frequently employed.

3.1. Collagen gels

Collagens represent the most abundant type of proteins in mammals making up to 35% of the whole body protein content. They are found in fibrillar and non-fibrillar forms and are widely distributed among tissues with a distinct structural, organizational and density variance among tissues and organs. Currently, 28 types of collagen have been described that are known to be products of 49 different α-chain gene products [37]. Collagen gels are one of the first employed 3D culturing systems used to study cellular adhesion and migration in three-dimensional environment [17, 38]. Currently collagen gels have found application in a wide variety of studies in the field of cellular motility [11] and the importance of physical parameters such as density, stiffness and elasticity for cellular adhesion, proliferation, migration and contraction [39]. Fibroblast cells, seeded in collagen gels, have been shown to acquire different morphology when compared to fibroblasts grown on two-dimensional surfaces and appear similar to their counterparts in normal connective tissue. The three-dimensional environment of the gel mimics the in vivo conditions and also causes normal polarization and differentiation of epithelial cells [16]. It has also been developed as a model for studying the progression of prostate and breast cancer [40, 41].

Few types of collagen gels are most widely employed as three-dimensional culturing systems. Pure gels that remain attached to the dish after polymerization are considered as "stressed". The cells plated within this 3D environment usually exert isometric tension. If the gels are released, detached from the bottom of the Petri dish, they contract and represent the so called "relaxed and loaded" gels. If the gels are detached from the dish before cells are being seeded, they represent "relaxed and unloaded" gels. The ease of manipulation of the collagen gel's stiffness provides a useful tool for the evaluation of the role of isometric tension for cell survival and differentiation as well as for the investigation of mechanical features of the environment and it's reorganization during wound healing processes or various pathological conditions [39]. Some interesting features of cell migration in 3D have been established using those different types of collagen gels. Migration in softer substrates, or compliant matrices, results in migratory activity that is independent of the small GTPase Rho [39], thus, the cell acquires an amoeboid phenotype. As tension increases and the extracellular matrix becomes more rigid, the migratory mode of fibroblasts switches over to Rho dependent migration [42] with a mesenchymal phenotype. Moreover, in order for fibroblasts to differentiate to myofibroblasts upon TGFβ stimulation, a typical process during wound healing, increased tension in the extracellular matrix is required [43]. Reorganization of the extracellular matrix also appears to be dependent on the mechanical properties of the substrate as incorporation of fibronectin in the extracellular matrix requires internal tension of the ECM [44].

Collagen gel-based dressings were also used in some of the first attempts to create in vitro equivalents of full thickness skin for regenerative medicine and tissue engineering applications

[45]. Currently there are a few temporary and semi-permanent dressings available as off-the-shelf products, intended for use as bioconstructs for skin reconstruction [46].

3.2. Fibrin gels

Fibrin gels are another type of easily manufactured 3D culturing systems. They are formed as a result of thrombin cleavage of fibrinogen, resulting in a mesh of fibrin fibers. Stressed, relaxed and loaded and relaxed and unloaded types of fibrin gels are also frequently used model systems. In normal physiological conditions fibrin represents the provisional matrix of the clot, formed after wounding. Thus, the defined use of fibrin gels to study cellular invasion and contraction during the processes of wound healing [47] has emerged. Historically, polymerized fibrin gels were one of the first scaffolds used for skin tissue engineering after severe burns or for treatment of chronic wounds [48]. Currently fibrin gels have found further applications in the field of vascular tissue engineering and are being extensively studied especially as a possible resolution of a number of rapidly growing problems related to arterial occlusive diseases [49]. Studies in cardiac tissue engineering and cartilage regeneration and reconstruction have also benefited of the use of this natural, biodegradable scaffold [50, 51].

3.3. Hyaluronan gels

Hyaluronan or hyaluronic acid is widely distributed throughout all tissues glycosaminoglycan. It is an anionic, nonsulfated polysaccharide, formed on the plasma membrane instead of in the Golgi apparatus, with molecular weight varying between 5 kDa and 2,000 kDa. Hyaluronan is a major component of the cartilage, synovial fluid, the extracellular matrix of the skin and has a major role during the developmental processes [52]. Presumably, due to the high abundance of the molecule and its role during development, wound healing and migration, hyaluronan gels became another suitable three-dimensional model for studies in numerous fields.

As a natural component of the cartilage, hyaluronan is being used as a milieu for culturing chondrocytes in vitro. Current research indicates that culturing in tissue-like hyaluronic 3D environment sustains chondrocytes phenotype, leading to increased proliferation, sulphated glycosaminoglycans production as well as collagen type II and aggrecan synthesis and indeed supports chondrogenic differentiation [53]. Additional studies have shown promising results concerning the use of hyaluronan for cartilage repair and as scaffold for regenerative medicine [54-56]. Another intriguing direction of studies is the utilization of three-dimensional hyaluronic acid scaffolds for culturing mesenchymal stem cells. Promising results from culturing stem cells in three-dimensional hyaluronan-based scaffolds have been obtained in regard to the generation of cartilage-like tissue for the use of regenerative medicine [57]. Hyaluronic acid gels have been also investigated as possible 3D scaffolds for culturing cardiomyocytes and hepatocytes in vitro [58, 59]. Therapeutical use of hyaluronan gels has been reported also in the field of adipose tissue engineering [60] as well as in neuromedicine. The use of this biodegradable material has revealed promising results in cell and drug delivery to the central nervous system[61].

3.4. Basement membrane extract gels

Almost 30 years ago the Engelbreth-Holm-Swarm (EHS) mouse sarcoma cell line was found to secrete vast amount of unknown protein mixture. Later it was determined that this mixture was composed of the typical for the basement membrane proteins collagen IV, laminin, entactin and the heparansulfate proteoglycan [62]. Further components like matrix metallo-proteinases as well as number of growth factors were also identified in this complex mixture. This protein composite is marketed by BD Biosciences under the trade name Matrigel®, but similar products are available from other sources. Matrigel resembles the complex extracellular matrix found in many tissues and is thus used by cell biologists as a substrate for cell culturing.

Utilization of the basement membrane matrix led to numerous scientific discoveries. For the first time the EHS matrix was used as a substrate to cultivate Sertoli cells, which led to their survival and the differentiation of the accompanying germ cells[63]. The first in vitro myeli-nation was also observed in cultures based on the basement membrane matrix. Carey et al. demonstrated in 1986 that rat Schwann cells cultured in 3D conditions based on basement membrane matrix show increased dendrite outgrowth and myelination [64]. Thus a reliable in vitro model for investigation of nerve regeneration was established.

Another interesting observation was made when epithelial and endothelial cells were cultured on basement membrane matrix. Both cell types show different morphology compared to flat 2D surfaces, but also form specific structures depending on whether cells are cultured on top or within the matrix. Ducts were formed when epithelial cells were cultured on top of the matrix, and acinar-like structures appeared when cells were embedded within the BME gel [65, 66]. Different types of acinar epithelial cells (breast epithelial cells, salivary gland cells, pancreatic and prostate cells) form distinct structures in 3D indeed clearly supporting the importance of the extracellular matrix in cellular differentiation and proliferation. Endothelial cells form capillary-like structures when seeded in lower counts, or monolayers when seeded in higher counts. These observations made possible the development of in vitro models for studying angiogenesis. Tumor-induced angiogenesis is a key prerequisite for neoplastic progression thus angiogenesis suppression is one of the major directions investigated as possible cancer treatment. Vascular endothelial cells form capillary-like structures when plated on 3D basement membrane gels and have provided a suitable model for testing pharmacological substances and screening of chemical agents as angiogenic inhibitors [67].

Basement membrane extract gels provided also another important model system aimed at investigation of cancer invasion and metastasis. Kramer et al. noticed that normal, non-malignant cells polarize on top of the matrix whereas malignant cells invaded the 3D basement membrane [68]. While normal cells attached, polarized and differentiated on top of the matrix and showed almost no migratory tendency, malignant cells exhibited increased invasive and migratory phenotype within the matrix. Formation of long protrusions in the direction of migration and channels of degraded matrix behind the cells were observed. Evidently, malignant cells mimicked their in vivo invasive behaviour since synthesis of proteolitic enzymes and degradation of the basement membrane are key events during tumor metastasis. Continuous investigation led to the development and improvement of invasion and metastasis assays [69, 70] providing identical conditions and criteria to measure the invasiveness of tumors and the efficiency of treatment.

Maybe one of the most significant discoveries related to the progress of regenerative medicine and tissue engineering is the possibility to culture stem cells on basement membrane matrix [71]. Normally the basement membrane is the first ECM to be synthesized in the developing embryo [72] hence the logical use for culturing stem cells. Feeder layers of irradiated mouse embryonic fibroblasts were required for long term culturing and limited the large scale production of human embryonic stem cells. Moreover, they present the possibility of viral cross contaminations. Utilization of other extracellular matrix components like fibronectin, collagen I, collagen IV or artificial substrates has failed to support undifferentiated stem cells growth [73], whereas coating of the dish with BME extract retained the undifferentiated state of human embryonic stem cells for up to 30 passages, maintaining their proliferation rate, high telomerase activity, normal karyotype and the expression of the pluripotency markers.

3.5. Cell-derived matrices

The use of three-dimensional gels of collagen, fibrin, basement membrane matrix or glycosa-minoglycans represents a significant advance in cell culturing. Those gels provide the much needed dimensionality to bring the environmental conditions closer to the in vivo settings. A major disadvantage of those models though is the fact that they still lack the chemical complexity and spatial organization of the ECM, characteristic for tissues (Figure 1). Indeed cells plated in three-dimensional gels degrade and reorganize to some extent the constituents of their surroundings and also secrete and integrate new components within the existing extracellular matrix [74]. Presumably cells are trying to shape their environment by their liking, but all those processes are believed to keep cells in an "activated" state that is unnatural for healthy tissue. In the quest for creating better model systems that approximate closer to different healthy tissues a few groups have developed during the last few decades affordable methods for creating cell derived three-dimensional cultures and matrices [9, 75-79]. Those methods are based on in vitro preparation of three-dimensional extracellular matrices made by the cells themselves. The result is a naturally synthesized and organized extracellular matrix, providing in vivo-like conditions.

Conducted research, based on these tissue-like cultures has already demonstrated significant differences between cells grown in three-dimensional cell derived matrices and other 3D culturing methods. Ahlfors and Billiar [79] demonstrated that culturing fibroblasts in appro-priate conditions induces synthesis of extracellular matrix components, thus resulting in a multilayer culture, with mechanical properties approximating normal tissue. Investigation of the mechanical properties of these cell derived 3D cultures revealed that the resulting matrices are stronger than collagen or fibrin 3D cultures. Moreover cells in naturally synthesized cultures had higher protein synthesis rate than fibroblasts cultured in collagen or fibrin gels, and more importantly, inhibition of collagen synthesis was not observed at later stages of cultivation. The production of matrices was achieved in serum supplemented media as well as in chemically defined media. The second option makes exploitation of this method relatively

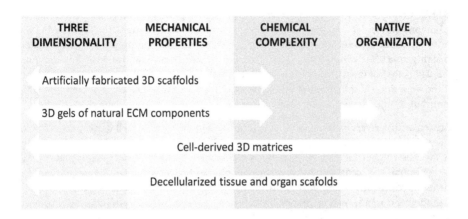

Figure 1. Schematic presentation of the main characteristics of 3D cell culture systems. While artificially fabricated 3D scaffolds can be designed with specific three dimensional organization and desired mechanical properties, they, however, generally lack the chemical complexity of the natural ECM. This limitation can be compensated to a certain extent by incorporation of natural ECM proteins or their peptides (indicated by additional small arrow). 3D gels, made out of natural ECM components have also restricted chemical complexity and in addition their structural organization is a result of spontaneous, rather than cell-directed polymerization. Cell-derived 3D matrices and decellularized tissues and organs meet the general requirements for in vivo-like 3D environment. However, they often pose difficulties in preparation and restrictions in their mass production (see text for details).

expensive, but increases the chances of utilization of such cultures for the needs of tissue engineering by greatly diminishing the possibilities of species or viral cross contamination.

As we have previously discussed, cellular morphology of fibroblasts differs between 2D and 3D conditions. Even though fibroblasts appear to acquire the same morphology when plated on collagen gels and cell derived matrices, there are a number of issues to be considered – fibroblasts attach, proliferate and migrate at much higher rate in cell derived matrices compared to collagen gels [9]. Though dimensionality influences fibroblast morphology one must also take into account the heterogeneity and specific organization of the extracellular matrix which are of significant importance as well. The fact that 3D matrix adhesions were established in cell derived extracellular matrices, but not in fibrin or collagen gels, or 2D surfaces coated with ECM components [9] supports the notion of the importance of structural organization of the environment. Both, the components and their colocalization in these adhesion structures differ from focal and fibrillar adhesions. Formation of such in vivo-like adhesions appears to depend on the heterogeneity and organization of the ECM and their formation does not require de novo protein synthesis during cellular adhesion. Major differences in signal transduction of fibroblasts in cell derived matrices were also discovered. The focal adhesion kinase (FAK), a molecule with exceptionally important role for cellular adhesion in conventional monolayer cultures, appears to be bypassed in in vivo-like conditions [8, 9]. In spite of this, downstream molecules maintain or even augment their activities, resulting in increased proliferation for example. Furthermore culturing of fibroblasts as a cell derived, three-dimensional multilayer culture leads to altered distribution of plasma membrane lipids

[80-82]. Changes of the localization and properties of plasma membrane cholesterol and sphingomyelin in 3D are a probable cause for lowered oxidative stress, thus supporting the growing number of studies indicating that 2D cultures are an inappropriate, stressful method for cultivation of cells. Moreover the differences in the structural organization of the membrane coupled with the higher content of cholesterol and sphingomyelin, the major lipid components of the lipid rafts, in the plasma membranes of cells in 3D tissue-like environment, probably contribute to the differences in cell signalling.

The major difference between other 3D culturing systems and the cell derived in vivo-like three-dimensional matrices is the fact that their ECM is synthesized and organized naturally by the cells. In vivo, the extracellular matrix main functions are to present proper and specific 3D environment to cells and thus to define boundaries between different tissues. It provides the required elasticity and integrity during tissue and organ development, but is also being degraded and remodelled during both developmental processes and disease. Serving as an adhesive substrate, the ECM directs migratory cells and variations in its components concentrations may act as chemotactic gradient as well as differences in its mechanical properties can serve as durotactic gradient. The extracellular matrix also participates in the accumulation, storage, release and presentation of growth factors to the cells. The synthesis and immobilization of growth factors is spatially and temporally regulated by the ECM and the release of the incorporated ligands is also dependent upon appropriate cell-mediated forces, proteolitic degradation and proper presentation to cells. As a supportive structure, the ECM also participates in the reciprocal mechanical signalling. The transmittion of forces to and by the cells is regulated by their mechanical receptors – the integrins – and is manifested by changes in the intracellular signalling resulting in activation of the cytoskeleton machinery, growth factor production, proliferation rate alteration, etc. [83]. Among all these specific characteristic of the extracellular matrix probably the most important one is the fact that it is a dynamic structure, being constantly remodelled by cells in response to intrinsic signals, depending on the specific periods of organism's development or due to occurring diseases.

Currently cell-derived extracellular matrices are being applied with great success for in vitro investigation of developmental processes [84], tumor cell invasion and the role of the accompanying stroma cells [85], the mechanisms of fibrosis [86], studies of cellular migration [12, 87], as drug screening systems [88], for exploring the processes of wound healing [78] and numerous other applications. Despite the advantages of this model system, there are still a lot of considerable hindrances for its application in regenerative medicine and tissue engineering. Therefore numerous groups have undertaken a "reverse" approach towards meeting the requirements of modern medicine (see below).

3.6. Decellularized tissues and organs as scaffolds for tissue engineering

The need for organ transplantation in modern society far much exceeds the donor availability. Moreover the immunological incompatibility limits further the patient's possibilities for finding a matching donor for the subsequent transplantation. Even if all those criteria are met more often than not, patients are treated with powerful immunosupressants to reduce the chances of transplant rejection.

The aspiring role of the ECM in governing the appropriate behaviour of a number of cell types led to the investigation of the properties and possible use in regenerative medicine of decellularized organs. The diversity of the extracellular matrix, its structure and micro-patterns suggest that specific cell types would overall "feel and perform better" if embedded in their corresponding natural matrix. There is a growing number of research to confirm this view. Culturing of hepatocytes as conventional monolayers, outside of their natural environment, results in loss of specific hepatocyte functions thus limiting the possibilities for their use in regenerative medicine. However, culturing of human hepatocytes in porcine liver-derived extracellular matrix supports albumin secretion and ammonia metabolism as well as restoration of hepatic transport activity [89]. Characteristic extracellular matrix is even required for the differentiation of human or murine embryonic stem cells to pneumocytes [90]. To date a number of ECM derived scaffolds have been described and investigated for use as organ reproducing systems, including heart-derived ECM [91], liver-derived ECM [92] and lung-derived ECM [93].

The process of removal of cells from the organ and obtaining a cell-free scaffold is crucial for preserving the scaffold's qualities and usually includes several stages. Physical methods, involving freezing and thawing, mechanical agitation and sonication, could be considered non-harmful to the remaining biological scaffold and are usually combined with enzymatic and/or chemical methods, depending on the organ that is being decellularized. Treatment with exo-and endonucleases yields better results than physical methods, but is likely to affect the extracellular matrix as well. Harsh chemical treatment with acid or alkaline solutions, especially detergents, either ionic or non-ionic, is known to extract cells from the extracellular matrix, but also severely damages the remaining scaffold. Depending on the organ, its cellular content, overall lipid content, ECM biochemical composition, structure and complexity an appropriate method for decellularization has to be selected. More often than not a combination of methods is used to achieve better results. Successful removal of cells would ideally yield DNA- and cell debris-free extracellular matrix that is not affected or altered by the applied treatments, thus resulting in a minimal or even absent immunological reaction towards the allogenic or xenogenic extracellular matrix. Some protocols have already been developed and successfully used for producing biological scaffolds for heart, liver and lung [91-93].

Decellularization of organs would ultimately provide the most suitable scaffold for reconstruction of an organ – a natural extracellular matrix. Repopulation with cells of the obtained scaffold is a process which also poses some difficulties in organ reconstruction. Reintroduction of cells to such scaffold requires organ-specific types of cells as well as endothelial and epithelial cells for rebuilding of blood vessels, stem or progenitor type of cells to support future cell renewal in the organ and most of all, distinct methods for introduction of the appropriate cell types to their targeted environment. When possible, autologous cells are used since they are less likely to provoke immune response and be rejected. Such cells also present lesser chance of inducing cancer or the possible non-immune toxic reactions caused by immunosupressants [94]. Allogenic cells from matching donors could also be used for regenerative purposes when autologus cells cannot be harvested, or are terminally damaged. Although these cells are not derived from the patient, they have some advantages too. The required cell types can be derived from healthy individuals, characterized and maintained until needed, thereby providing the opportunity for faster therapy application. A well known example of such use of allogenic cells is provided by the mesenchymal bone marrow cells.

Often isolation of highly proliferating autologous cells from most organs is an almost impossible task. The use of embryonic stem cells could help solve this problem but the employment of human embryonic stem cells is still bounded up with heated moral debates. In addition it is a quite expensive technology, demanding proven methods for directed differentiation and extensive clinical trials. Therefore the use of adult cells with similar properties emerged as possible solution. Adult stem cells represent autologus cells which are multipotent and capable of self-renew. They have been known to exist in number of tissues like the gonads, intestine, skin and blood, and further data indicates their presence in adipose tissue [95], kidney [96], lung [97] and muscle [98]. In recent years, scientists have tried to identify specific markers to ease the isolation of adult stem cells, but such insignia are yet to be defined for most of them. Furthermore, it is currently evident that adult stem cells are localized in a specific extracellular environment – their niche. Signalling to and regulation of the self-renewal or differentiation processes appears to be tightly linked to the stem cell's niche, suggesting that micro-environmental cues may also be regulating cellular "stemness" [99]. A possible localization of different types of adult stem cells in niches in close proximity also exists [100, 101]. Thus, even though the specific localization of diverse types of adult stem cells have been identified, their isolation and further characterisation has proven to be an extremely difficult task. Label retention techniques and in vivo linage tracing as well as in vitro culturing and transplantation have yielded promising results and have aided the significant advancement in the field, but isolation of adult stem cells is still a major difficulty [99]. Despite the obstacles though, different types of adult stem cells have already found application in regenerative medicine [57, 102-104].

As pointed above, harvesting highly proliferating cells from healthy tissues has rendered a difficult task. Therefore researchers have sought to develop novel technologies that would aid obtaining and multiplication of such cells for further use in regenerative medicine. A promising technique developed just a few years ago is the induction of pluripotency in differentiated somatic cells. In 2006 Takahashi and Yamanaka introduced a method for inducing pluripotency in fibroblast cells by overexpression of four transcript factors – Oct-4, c-Myc, Sox2 and Klf4 [105]. Their results showed that the timed overexpression of these factors is sufficient to convert fibroblasts to embryonic stem cell-like cells, termed induced pluripotent stem cells (iPSC), with many subsequent articles confirming their observations. The iPS cells are able to differentiate to any type of cell, just like embryonic stem cells, but since the progenitor cells are derived from the adult organism their use is liberated from the moral burdens concerning the use of embryonic stem cells. Research indicates that the genetic profile of good quality iPSC and embryonic stem cells is nearly identical, although some articles suggest that there may be some differences, probably attributed to different laboratory practices [106-108]. Further analysis of the whole genome have indeed found 71 differently methylated regions between iPSC and embryonic stem cells and 2,179 between iPSC and fibroblast [109], supporting the hypothesis that probably even though somatic cells are converted to pluripotent cells, there is still a "memory" preserved of the type of the donor cell.

Even though there are a lot of difficulties with the production of iPS cells, already a plethora of articles has demonstrated the ability of iPS cells to differentiate to numerous types of cells, thus providing the ability to direct the in vitro differentiation of iPS cells to the required cell type for the specific therapy. Moreover significant results have been accomplished, namely the generation of adult mice from iPS cells [110] thus confirming the vast capabilities of such cells. Therapeutically, iPS cells have been used together with gene therapy to correct genetic defects in mice, with two studies already showing promising results in the treatment of different types of anaemia [111, 112]. Future efforts in the field of iPS cells though have to be made before a successful iPSC therapy for human patients becomes a reality – research is currently targeted towards the development of methods of pluripotency induction, not relying on viral transduction, therefore lowering the possibility of cancer induction by the transplanted iPS cells as well as improvement of the efficacy of reprogramming. Furthermore the remaining questions of whether the donor cells are completely reprogrammed or retain a "memory" of their differentiated state are still to be answered.

4. Does a perfect 3D system exist?

In vitro 3D models present the opportunity to investigate in depth the molecular mechanisms of the interactions between cells and the extracellular matrix. The increased number of research based on 3D scaffolds, mimicking specific physiological and developmental processes, as well as tissues, bridges the gap between laboratory investigation and unimpeded tissue regeneration. At the same time the increasing number of research has made it clear that variables such as cell source, the extracellular matrix's biochemical and mechanical properties, growth factor cues and developmental stage affect cell behavior and therapy outcome, imposing the need of even more careful reconsideration of yet the slightly interfering environmental factors for the successful outcome of regenerative therapies or tissue engineering.

Development of optimal bioengineered scaffolds requires indepth knowledge of physiology and understanding of cell–cell and cell–ECM interactions. The choice of inappropriate model system could have a negative effect on the study or the therapy outcome. Such an example could be any of the discussed 3D culturing systems. Sometimes even slight changes in experimental design like difference in cell count in collagen gels for example could lead to different migrational patterns [87] or as mentioned, the change of the substrate stiffness can induce different responses of cells to the environment [14]. Still, the obscured causes underlying such different outcomes are yet to be defined. Another example could be the inappropriate use of three-dimensional BME gels. In vivo basement membranes represent thin extracellular structures that underlie endothelial and epithelial structures. Basement membranes also surround muscle, fat and nerve cells. Moreover the composition and the amount of the basement membrane are specific and vary in different tissues and during particular stages of development. Even though introduction of cells to a 3D environment, based on basement membrane matrix, results in numerous morphological and physiological changes, there are a number of discrepancies to be considered and questions to be answered:

- Contact with the basement membrane is not typical for all cell types, but a lot of cells express receptors for components of the basement membrane matrix. Therefore what would happen with cells that accidentally get caught in such unnatural environment? Would they become apoptotic or would they transform into malignant cells?

- Not all cell types respond to the basement membrane matrix and thus an optimization of the environment is required.

- Differences in basement membrane matrix composition during development imply that cells may respond to the matrix up to a certain stage. Acquisition and synchronization of cells of developmentally correct phases could be difficult and thus could inappropriately selected cells lead to activation of pathologic-like processes?

- The available basement membrane extract is of cancerous origin. Since tumor environment has been shown to be sufficient to promote desmoplastic differentiation [85] is it possible that contact of normal cells with cancerous cell-derived BME could induce their transformation?

All these discrepancies and unanswered questions do not make the BME gels unsuitable model systems, but stress the importance of experimental design. Hakkinen et al. have shown that normal fibroblasts respond unexpectedly in 3D BME gels – they acquire a rounded morphology with short protrusions, possibly for environmental sensing and do not migrate [12] – behavior typical for non-malignant fibroblasts, thus supporting the notion that an adequate model should be chosen for each experimental design. Indeed BME gels provide scientists with a great tool to study malignant cell invasion through the basement membrane [70, 113], with numerous assays developed for investigation of the mechanisms of invasion. Moreover comparison between different three-dimensional scaffolds in terms of cell morphology, adhesion and migration and cytoskeletal organization concluded that indeed careful attention should be paid on the experimental design [12].

Use of other types of 3D gels faces researchers with similar problems. Neither collagen nor fibrin or hyaluronan gels incorporate other components of connective tissue. They are suitable for investigation of a specific response of a specific cell type towards distinctively modulated environments, but are still far away from the complex organization of the native extracellular environment. At the same time the provisional matrix of a blood clot is formed of disorganized fibrin mesh, just like the in vitro 3D gels. Cell-derived matrices on the other hand represent a complex, cell-organized structure based on cell-specific type of expressed matrix components. However, it is possible that in vitro generated cell derived matrices could also have different matrix composition, pore sizes, mechanical and biochemical characteristics than in vivo analogues because of the initially unnatural substrate cells were cultured on. Thus it is important of one to consider the specific characteristic of the tissue in vivo or the nature of the modeled process in order to be able to select an appropriate 3D matrix for in vitro research or for in vitro based preparation for therapies.

Besides looking at the ECM as a 3D structure one must not forget that in vivo cells do have a specific polarity that is usually lost during conventional 2D cultivation, and sometimes even in 3D, if an inappropriate environment has been selected. Fibroblasts for example, lack an apical and basal organization in vivo. So when placed back in 3D environment after being cultured as 2D monolayers they tend to regain their typical in vivo morphology [9, 74, 114], but the essence of the environment also has to be considered since it could provoke different morphology [12]. Moreover, both the mechanical and the structural state of the environment have to be taken into consideration. Recent studies have shown that gene expression patterns, fibroblast morphology, as well as organization of the extracellular environment differ not only between particular healthy tissues but also compared to tumor stroma [85, 115, 116]. Furthermore it is currently evident that cells do feel and respond in different ways to the environment – fibroblast cells differentiate to myofibroblasts due to changes in the substrate stiffness [86] and begin to remodel the extracellular matrix. Stem cells have the ability to differentiate to osteogenic, myoblastic and neuronal lineages based just on the change on substrate stiffness [13]. Tumor associated stroma alone was shown to be able to induce desmoplastic stroma fibroblast differentiation [85] as well as at later stages of tumor progression, to be more permissive for epithelial invasion [117]. Taking into consideration these differences it is not surprising that the compliance of the substrate and its topography and mechanical features can control cellular behavior. Therefore the transplantation of cells into bioengineered scaffolds for the purposes of regenerative medicine or tissue engineering has to be precisely assessed and executed, since even the small differences in the substrate's composition, organization or stiffness have the potential to alter the donor cells gene expression [85, 118] or to promote tumorigenic transformation [119].

Despite the drawbacks revealed about each type of bioengineered scaffolds they have already found use in regenerative medicine. Fibrin and collagen grafts for example were among the first used in burn patients for skin reconstruction. Study by Chua et al. has shown that use of skin tissue constructs has reduced mortality in patients with 60% of total body area burns from 100% in 1952 to 41,4% in 2003 [120]. The advance in the skin tissue regeneration is accentuated by the high number of currently available off-the-shelf bioengineered skin grafts [46], that could be grouped by several criteria:

- Biomaterial – biological (autologus, allogenic and xenogenic) and synthetic (biodegradable, non-biodegradable)

- Duration of the graft – permanent, semi-permanent, temporary

- Composition regarding cell content – cellularized or acellular

- Anatomical structure – epidermal, dermal, composite

Together with this immense success in the field of burn wounds and the increase in survival rate though, patients are faced with new obstacles. More often than not wounds in surviving patients develop severe fibrosis after healing. The resulting hypertrophic scars present a major discomfort in survivor's life by possibly limiting the range of motion of joints, also resulting in impaired thermal regulation and not at the least a disturbed visual appearance [121].

In spite of the advances made in skin tissue engineering and without undervaluing the accomplished results there is still a lot of progress to be made towards the prefect reconstruction of the skin. There still isn't an available option that makes possible the regeneration of hair follicles and sebatious glands, thus allowing for rehabilitation of thermal regulation. Even though the perfect skin graft is still to be created, the available skin models have made a significant impact in in vitro studies regarding skin biology and skin disease progression: engineered skin of different aspects helps in producing more relevant results than 2D cultures, thus leading to reduced use of animals for experimentation. As discussed earlier investigation of cell–cell and cell–extracellular matrix interactions has evolved rapidly due to the use of skin tissue-mimicking models. Wound healing, skin contraction [122] and angiogenesis are all fields benefiting from the use of 3D skin equivalents. Investigation of skin diseases such as melanoma invasion [123, 124], psoriasis [125] and skin blistering disorders [126] is also making significant progress based on engineered skin.

Besides skin tissue engineering biological scaffolds have found use in other sections of tissue engineering. Promising results are obtained with decellularization and recellularization of heart, liver and lungs. After recellularization of a hearth-derived ECM, a macroscopic contraction and pump function of the newly generated heart were observed in vitro [91] – indeed a promising result for the generation of a biological artificial heart. Recellularization of liver [92] and lungs [127] has gone even further and transplantation of the newly formed organs back to animals showed that they are able to sustain their natural functions. Probably one of the highest successes of tissue engineering for regenerative medicine is the successful transplant of trachea in a 30-year old patient [128] based on decellularized tracheal scaffold, reseeded with autologus epithelial and mesenchymal cells thus reducing the possibility of organ rejection and the need of strong immunosupressants. Despite the great success in the field the major disadvantage of these scaffolds still persists – the need of a donor organ for their preparation. Nevertheless the first successful transplantation of entirely bioengineered constructs, a completely new tracheobronchial tube in a patient suffering from tracheal cancer, is already a reality, partly due to the virtue to three-dimensional model systems [129].

Based on the review of decades of research it is currently evident that a perfect 3D system able to fulfill all scientific and medicinal requirements does not exist. On the contrary – a careful and differential approach towards appropriate 3D system selection, experimental or therapeutical design and data interpretation is required for every particular case (Figure 2). Such approach would contribute to the optimal outcome of the specific therapy or the distinct experiment thus leading the way to unimpeded regenerative medicine.

5. Conclusion

The evolution of the cell culturing method has led to the sophistication of culturing procedures with one main goal – to approximate in vitro conditions to in vivo. The advancement of three-dimensional culturing models has allowed for an in depth understanding of cellular behavior and especially the role of the cell's environment has emerged as an important modulator of cellular functions. Current data has made it clear that future development and use of superior three-dimensional cultures should focus not just on the dimensionality of the environment per se, but mainly on its characteristics – biochemical composition, production source and possible unwanted cell-cueing signals, mechanical properties, etc. thus making 3D culturing, along with regenerative medicine multidisciplinary fields. However, as science advances, more and more questions emerge and await answers in order to confirm the long term safety of the applied methods for human therapy.

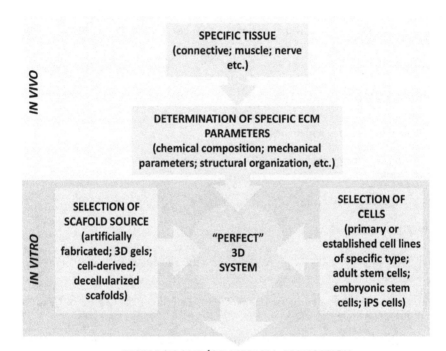

Figure 2. General strategy for design of a "perfect" 3D system. The specific set of ECM characteristics, typical for selected normal tissue can be determined. Based on these studies, a scaffold with matching parameters and suitable cells can be identified and combined in vitro for development of particular, tailored made 3D culture, meeting the needs of a specific research or specific therapy.

During the resolution of the moral issues concerning the use of human embryonic stem cells or donor organs the remaining fields continue to advance rapidly. It appears that isolation of autologus cells, their expansion in vitro and probably stimulation to produce extracellular matrix with the required dimensionality, biochemical and mechanical properties would represent the optimal tissue engineered scaffold for tissue and organ reconstruction. Further advance in the field of regenerative medicine and tissue engineering would possibly see the development of 4D model systems, incorporating time as the forth dimension. Such models would represent not just single stages of organ development or disease, but the chronology of their maturation/progression, thus providing an opportunity to transfer developmental processes to in vitro conditions.

Acknowledgements

This publication is supported with funding form Grant № ДДВУ02/9 by the National Science Fund

Author details

Aleksandar Evangelatov and Roumen Pankov

Department of Cytology, Histology and Embryology, Sofia University "St. Kliment Ohridski", Sofia, Bulgaria

References

[1] Hamburger V. Wilhelm Roux: visionary with a blind spot. J Hist Biol 1997;30(2) 229-38.

[2] Carrel A. On the Permanent Life of Tissues Outside of the Organism. J Exp Med 1912;15(5) 516-28.

[3] Eagle H. Nutrition needs of mammalian cells in tissue culture. Science 1955;122(3168) 501-14.

[4] Scherer WF, Syverton JT, Gey GO. Studies on the propagation in vitro of poliomyelitis viruses. IV. Viral multiplication in a stable strain of human malignant epithelial cells (strain HeLa) derived from an epidermoid carcinoma of the cervix. J Exp Med 1953;97(5) 695-710.

[5] Martin GR. Isolation of a pluripotent cell line from early mouse embryos cultured in medium conditioned by teratocarcinoma stem cells. Proc Natl Acad Sci U S A 1981;78(12) 7634-8.

[6] Evans MJ, Kaufman MH. Establishment in culture of pluripotential cells from mouse embryos. Nature 1981;292(5819) 154-6.

[7] Thomson JA, Itskovitz-Eldor J, Shapiro SS, Waknitz MA, Swiergiel JJ, Marshall VS, et al. Embryonic stem cell lines derived from human blastocysts. Science 1998;282(5391) 1145-7.

[8] Damianova R, Stefanova N, Cukierman E, Momchilova A, Pankov R. Three-dimensional matrix induces sustained activation of ERK1/2 via Src/Ras/Raf signaling pathway. Cell Biol Int 2008;32(2) 229-34.

[9] Cukierman E, Pankov R, Stevens DR, Yamada KM. Taking cell-matrix adhesions to the third dimension. Science 2001;294(5547) 1708-12.

[10] Geiger B, Bershadsky A, Pankov R, Yamada KM. Transmembrane crosstalk between the extracellular matrix--cytoskeleton crosstalk. Nat Rev Mol Cell Biol 2001;2(11) 793-805.

[11] Friedl P, Brocker EB. The biology of cell locomotion within three-dimensional extracellular matrix. Cell Mol Life Sci 2000;57(1) 41-64.

[12] Hakkinen KM, Harunaga JS, Doyle AD, Yamada KM. Direct comparisons of the morphology, migration, cell adhesions, and actin cytoskeleton of fibroblasts in four different three-dimensional extracellular matrices. Tissue Eng Part A 2011;17(5-6) 713-24.

[13] Engler AJ, Sen S, Sweeney HL, Discher DE. Matrix elasticity directs stem cell lineage specification. Cell 2006;126(4) 677-89.

[14] Discher DE, Janmey P, Wang YL. Tissue cells feel and respond to the stiffness of their substrate. Science 2005;310(5751) 1139-43.

[15] Zamir E, Katz BZ, Aota S, Yamada KM, Geiger B, Kam Z. Molecular diversity of cell-matrix adhesions. J Cell Sci 1999;112 (Pt 11) 1655-69.

[16] Barcellos-Hoff MH, Aggeler J, Ram TG, Bissell MJ. Functional differentiation and alveolar morphogenesis of primary mammary cultures on reconstituted basement membrane. Development 1989;105(2) 223-35.

[17] Elsdale T, Bard J. Collagen substrata for studies on cell behavior. J Cell Biol 1972;54(3) 626-37.

[18] Trinh LA, Stainier DY. Fibronectin regulates epithelial organization during myocardial migration in zebrafish. Dev Cell 2004;6(3) 371-82.

[19] Ryan MC, Lee K, Miyashita Y, Carter WG. Targeted disruption of the LAMA3 gene in mice reveals abnormalities in survival and late stage differentiation of epithelial cells. J Cell Biol 1999;145(6) 1309-23.

[20] Liu X, Wu H, Byrne M, Jeffrey J, Krane S, Jaenisch R. A targeted mutation at the known collagenase cleavage site in mouse type I collagen impairs tissue remodeling. J Cell Biol 1995;130(1) 227-37.

[21] Wenstrup RJ, Florer JB, Brunskill EW, Bell SM, Chervoneva I, Birk DE. Type V collagen controls the initiation of collagen fibril assembly. J Biol Chem 2004;279(51) 53331-7.

[22] Wagenseil JE, Mecham RP. Vascular extracellular matrix and arterial mechanics. Physiol Rev 2009;89(3) 957-89.

[23] Arikawa-Hirasawa E, Watanabe H, Takami H, Hassell JR, Yamada Y. Perlecan is essential for cartilage and cephalic development. Nat Genet 1999;23(3) 354-8.

[24] Watanabe H, Kimata K, Line S, Strong D, Gao LY, Kozak CA, et al. Mouse cartilage matrix deficiency (cmd) caused by a 7 bp deletion in the aggrecan gene. Nat Genet 1994;7(2) 154-7.

[25] Martin-Belmonte F, Gassama A, Datta A, Yu W, Rescher U, Gerke V, et al. PTEN-mediated apical segregation of phosphoinositides controls epithelial morphogenesis through Cdc42. Cell 2007;128(2) 383-97.

[26] Kesavan G, Sand FW, Greiner TU, Johansson JK, Kobberup S, Wu X, et al. Cdc42-mediated tubulogenesis controls cell specification. Cell 2009;139(4) 791-801.

[27] Burridge K TS. Editorial overview: Cell-to-cell contact and extracellular matrix. Current Opinion in Cell Biology 2001(13) 525-8.

[28] Hynes RO. Cell adhesion: old and new questions. Trends Cell Biol 1999;9(12) M33-7.

[29] Inman JL, Bissell MJ. Apical polarity in three-dimensional culture systems: where to now? J Biol 2010;9(1) 2.

[30] Persidis A. Tissue engineering. Nat Biotechnol 1999;17(5) 508-10.

[31] Liu X, Won Y, Ma PX. Porogen-induced surface modification of nano-fibrous poly(L-lactic acid) scaffolds for tissue engineering. Biomaterials 2006;27(21) 3980-7.

[32] Liu X, Smith LA, Hu J, Ma PX. Biomimetic nanofibrous gelatin/apatite composite scaffolds for bone tissue engineering. Biomaterials 2009;30(12) 2252-8.

[33] Ozkan S, Kalyon DM, Yu X, McKelvey CA, Lowinger M. Multifunctional protein-encapsulated polycaprolactone scaffolds: fabrication and in vitro assessment for tissue engineering. Biomaterials 2009;30(26) 4336-47.

[34] Sun W, Lal P. Recent development on computer aided tissue engineering--a review. Comput Methods Programs Biomed 2002;67(2) 85-103.

[35] Zhang S, Zhao X. Design of molecular biological materials using peptide motifs. Journal of Materials Chemistry 2004;14(14) 2082-6.

[36] Li D, Xia Y. Electrospinning of Nanofibers: Reinventing the Wheel? Advanced Materials 2004;16(14) 1151-70.

[37] Gordon MK, Hahn RA. Collagens. Cell Tissue Res 2010;339(1) 247-57.

[38] Schor SL, Schor AM, Winn B, Rushton G. The use of three-dimensional collagen gels for the study of tumour cell invasion in vitro: experimental parameters influencing cell migration into the gel matrix. Int J Cancer 1982;29(1) 57-62.

[39] Grinnell F. Fibroblast-collagen-matrix contraction: growth-factor signalling and me-chanical loading. Trends Cell Biol 2000;10(9) 362-5.

[40] Petersen OW, Ronnov-Jessen L, Howlett AR, Bissell MJ. Interaction with basement membrane serves to rapidly distinguish growth and differentiation pattern of normal and malignant human breast epithelial cells. Proc Natl Acad Sci U S A 1992;89(19) 9064-8.

[41] Koutsilieris M, Sourla A, Pelletier G, Doillon CJ. Three-dimensional type I collagen gel system for the study of osteoblastic metastases produced by metastatic prostate cancer. J Bone Miner Res 1994;9(11) 1823-32.

[42] Parizi M, Howard EW, Tomasek JJ. Regulation of LPA-promoted myofibroblast con-traction: role of Rho, myosin light chain kinase, and myosin light chain phosphatase. Exp Cell Res 2000;254(2) 210-20.

[43] Vaughan MB, Howard EW, Tomasek JJ. Transforming growth factor-beta1 promotes the morphological and functional differentiation of the myofibroblast. Exp Cell Res 2000;257(1) 180-9.

[44] Halliday NL, Tomasek JJ. Mechanical properties of the extracellular matrix influence fibronectin fibril assembly in vitro. Exp Cell Res 1995;217(1) 109-17.

[45] Bell E, Ehrlich HP, Buttle DJ, Nakatsuji T. Living tissue formed in vitro and accepted as skin-equivalent tissue of full thickness. Science 1981;211(4486) 1052-4.

[46] Shevchenko RV, James SL, James SE. A review of tissue-engineered skin biocon-structs available for skin reconstruction. J R Soc Interface 2010;7(43) 229-58.

[47] Even-Ram S. Fibrin gel model for assessment of cellular contractility. Methods Mol Biol 2009;522 251-9.

[48] Horch RE, Bannasch H, Kopp J, Andree C, Stark GB. Single-cell suspensions of cul-tured human keratinocytes in fibrin-glue reconstitute the epidermis. Cell Transplant 1998;7(3) 309-17.

[49] Shaikh FM, Callanan A, Kavanagh EG, Burke PE, Grace PA, McGloughlin TM. Fi-brin: a natural biodegradable scaffold in vascular tissue engineering. Cells Tissues Organs 2008;188(4) 333-46.

[50] Yuan Ye K, Sullivan KE, Black LD. Encapsulation of cardiomyocytes in a fibrin hy-drogel for cardiac tissue engineering. J Vis Exp 2011(55).

[51] Chien CS, Ho HO, Liang YC, Ko PH, Sheu MT, Chen CH. Incorporation of exudates of human platelet-rich fibrin gel in biodegradable fibrin scaffolds for tissue engineer-ing of cartilage. J Biomed Mater Res B Appl Biomater 2012;100(4) 948-55.

[52] Fraser JR, Laurent TC, Laurent UB. Hyaluronan: its nature, distribution, functions and turnover. J Intern Med 1997;242(1) 27-33.

[53] Kang JY, Chung CW, Sung JH, Park BS, Choi JY, Lee SJ, et al. Novel porous matrix of hyaluronic acid for the three-dimensional culture of chondrocytes. Int J Pharm 2009;369(1-2) 114-20.

[54] Amini AA, Nair LS. Injectable hydrogels for bone and cartilage repair. Biomed Mater 2012;7(2) 024105.

[55] Pavesio A, Abatangelo G, Borrione A, Brocchetta D, Hollander AP, Kon E, et al. Hya-luronan-based scaffolds (Hyalograft C) in the treatment of knee cartilage defects: pre-liminary clinical findings. Novartis Found Symp 2003;249 203-17; discussion 29-33, 34-8, 39-41.

[56] Kon E, Filardo G, Tschon M, Fini M, Giavaresi G, Marchesini Reggiani L, et al. TIS-SUE ENGINEERING FOR TOTAL MENISCAL SUBSTITUTION. Animal study in sheep model: results at 12 months. Tissue Eng Part A 2012.

[57] Stok KS, Lisignoli G, Cristino S, Facchini A, Muller R. Mechano-functional assess-ment of human mesenchymal stem cells grown in three-dimensional hyaluronan-based scaffolds for cartilage tissue engineering. J Biomed Mater Res A 2010;93(1) 37-45.

[58] Yuan Ye K, Sullivan KE, Black LD. Encapsulation of cardiomyocytes in a fibrin hy-drogel for cardiac tissue engineering. J Vis Exp (55).

[59] Skardal A, Smith L, Bharadwaj S, Atala A, Soker S, Zhang Y. Tissue specific synthetic ECM hydrogels for 3-D in vitro maintenance of hepatocyte function. Biomaterials 2012;33(18) 4565-75.

[60] Young DA, Christman KL. Injectable biomaterials for adipose tissue engineering. Bi-omed Mater 2012;7(2) 024104.

[61] Pakulska MM, Ballios BG, Shoichet MS. Injectable hydrogels for central nervous sys-tem therapy. Biomed Mater 2012;7(2) 024101.

[62] Kleinman HK, McGarvey ML, Liotta LA, Robey PG, Tryggvason K, Martin GR. Isola-tion and characterization of type IV procollagen, laminin, and heparan sulfate pro-teoglycan from the EHS sarcoma. Biochemistry 1982;21(24) 6188-93.

[63] Hadley MA, Byers SW, Suarez-Quian CA, Kleinman HK, Dym M. Extracellular ma-trix regulates Sertoli cell differentiation, testicular cord formation, and germ cell de-velopment in vitro. J Cell Biol 1985;101(4) 1511-22.

[64] Carey DJ, Todd MS, Rafferty CM. Schwann cell myelination: induction by exogenous basement membrane-like extracellular matrix. J Cell Biol 1986;102(6) 2254-63.

[65] Li ML, Aggeler J, Farson DA, Hatier C, Hassell J, Bissell MJ. Influence of a reconsti-tuted basement membrane and its components on casein gene expression and secre-tion in mouse mammary epithelial cells. Proc Natl Acad Sci U S A 1987;84(1) 136-40.

[66] Kubota Y, Kleinman HK, Martin GR, Lawley TJ. Role of laminin and basement membrane in the morphological differentiation of human endothelial cells into capillary-like structures. J Cell Biol 1988;107(4) 1589-98.

[67] Benelli R, Albini A. In vitro models of angiogenesis: the use of Matrigel. Int J Biol Markers 1999;14(4) 243-6.

[68] Kramer RH, Bensch KG, Wong J. Invasion of reconstituted basement membrane matrix by metastatic human tumor cells. Cancer Res 1986;46(4 Pt 2) 1980-9.

[69] Albini A, Iwamoto Y, Kleinman HK, Martin GR, Aaronson SA, Kozlowski JM, et al. A rapid in vitro assay for quantitating the invasive potential of tumor cells. Cancer Res 1987;47(12) 3239-45.

[70] Albini A, Benelli R, Noonan DM, Brigati C. The "chemoinvasion assay": a tool to study tumor and endothelial cell invasion of basement membranes. Int J Dev Biol 2004;48(5-6) 563-71.

[71] Xu C, Inokuma MS, Denham J, Golds K, Kundu P, Gold JD, et al. Feeder-free growth of undifferentiated human embryonic stem cells. Nat Biotechnol 2001;19(10) 971-4.

[72] LeBleu VS, Macdonald B, Kalluri R. Structure and function of basement membranes. Exp Biol Med (Maywood) 2007;232(9) 1121-9.

[73] Hakala H, Rajala K, Ojala M, Panula S, Areva S, Kellomaki M, et al. Comparison of biomaterials and extracellular matrices as a culture platform for multiple, independently derived human embryonic stem cell lines. Tissue Eng Part A 2009;15(7) 1775-85.

[74] Grinnell F. Fibroblast biology in three-dimensional collagen matrices. Trends Cell Biol 2003;13(5) 264-9.

[75] Beacham DA, Amatangelo MD, Cukierman E. Preparation of extracellular matrices produced by cultured and primary fibroblasts. Curr Protoc Cell Biol 2007;Chapter 10 Unit 10 9.

[76] Grinnell F, Fukamizu H, Pawelek P, Nakagawa S. Collagen processing, crosslinking, and fibril bundle assembly in matrix produced by fibroblasts in long-term cultures supplemented with ascorbic acid. Exp Cell Res 1989;181(2) 483-91.

[77] Clark RA, McCoy GA, Folkvord JM, McPherson JM. TGF-beta 1 stimulates cultured human fibroblasts to proliferate and produce tissue-like fibroplasia: a fibronectin matrix-dependent event. J Cell Physiol 1997;170(1) 69-80.

[78] Ohgoda O, Sakai A, Koga H, Kanai K, Miyazaki T, Niwano Y. Fibroblast-migration in a wound model of ascorbic acid-supplemented three-dimensional culture system: the effects of cytokines and malotilate, a new wound healing stimulant, on cell-migration. J Dermatol Sci 1998;17(2) 123-31.

[79] Ahlfors JE, Billiar KL. Biomechanical and biochemical characteristics of a human fibroblast-produced and remodeled matrix. Biomaterials 2007;28(13) 2183-91.

[80] Stefanova N, Staneva G, Petkova D, Lupanova T, Pankov R, Momchilova A. Cell culturing in a three-dimensional matrix affects the localization and properties of plasma membrane cholesterol. Cell Biol Int 2009;33(10) 1079-86.

[81] Lupanova T, Stefanova N, Petkova D, Staneva G, Jordanova A, Koumanov K, et al. Alterations in the content and physiological role of sphingomyelin in plasma membranes of cells cultured in three-dimensional matrix. Mol Cell Biochem 2010;340(1-2) 215-22.

[82] Staneva G, Lupanova T, Chachaty C, Petkova D, Koumanov K, Pankov R, et al. Structural organization of plasma membrane lipids isolated from cells cultured as a monolayer and in tissue-like conditions. J Colloid Interface Sci 2011;359(1) 202-9.

[83] Rozario T, DeSimone DW. The extracellular matrix in development and morphogenesis: a dynamic view. Dev Biol 2010;341(1) 126-40.

[84] Onodera T, Sakai T, Hsu JC, Matsumoto K, Chiorini JA, Yamada KM. Btbd7 regulates epithelial cell dynamics and branching morphogenesis. Science 2010;329(5991) 562-5.

[85] Amatangelo MD, Bassi DE, Klein-Szanto AJ, Cukierman E. Stroma-derived three-dimensional matrices are necessary and sufficient to promote desmoplastic differentiation of normal fibroblasts. Am J Pathol 2005;167(2) 475-88.

[86] Hinz B. Tissue stiffness, latent TGF-beta1 activation, and mechanical signal transduction: implications for the pathogenesis and treatment of fibrosis. Curr Rheumatol Rep 2009;11(2) 120-6.

[87] Friedl P. Prespecification and plasticity: shifting mechanisms of cell migration. Curr Opin Cell Biol 2004;16(1) 14-23.

[88] Cukierman E, Bassi D. The mesenchymal tumor microenvironment: A drug resistant niche. Cell Adh Migr 2012;6(3) 285-96.

[89] Sellaro TL, Ranade A, Faulk DM, McCabe GP, Dorko K, Badylak SF, et al. Maintenance of human hepatocyte function in vitro by liver-derived extracellular matrix gels. Tissue Eng Part A 2010;16(3) 1075-82.

[90] Lin YM, Zhang A, Rippon HJ, Bismarck A, Bishop AE. Tissue engineering of lung: the effect of extracellular matrix on the differentiation of embryonic stem cells to pneumocytes. Tissue Eng Part A 2010;16(5) 1515-26.

[91] Ott HC, Matthiesen TS, Goh SK, Black LD, Kren SM, Netoff TI, et al. Perfusion-decellularized matrix: using nature's platform to engineer a bioartificial heart. Nat Med 2008;14(2) 213-21.

[92] Uygun BE, Soto-Gutierrez A, Yagi H, Izamis ML, Guzzardi MA, Shulman C, et al. Organ reengineering through development of a transplantable recellularized liver graft using decellularized liver matrix. Nat Med 2010;16(7) 814-20.

[93] Petersen TH, Calle EA, Zhao L, Lee EJ, Gui L, Raredon MB, et al. Tissue-engineered lungs for in vivo implantation. Science 2010;329(5991) 538-41.

[94] Benoit E, O'Donnell Jr TF, Patel AN. Safety and efficacy of autologous cell therapy in critical limb ischemia: a systematic review of the literature. Cell Transplant 2012.

[95] Baer PC, Geiger H. Adipose-derived mesenchymal stromal/stem cells: tissue localization, characterization, and heterogeneity. Stem Cells Int 2012;2012 812693.

[96] Oliver JA, Maarouf O, Cheema FH, Martens TP, Al-Awqati Q. The renal papilla is a niche for adult kidney stem cells. J Clin Invest 2004;114(6) 795-804.

[97] Kim CF, Jackson EL, Woolfenden AE, Lawrence S, Babar I, Vogel S, et al. Identification of bronchioalveolar stem cells in normal lung and lung cancer. Cell 2005;121(6) 823-35.

[98] Collins CA, Olsen I, Zammit PS, Heslop L, Petrie A, Partridge TA, et al. Stem cell function, self-renewal, and behavioral heterogeneity of cells from the adult muscle satellite cell niche. Cell 2005;122(2) 289-301.

[99] Snippert HJ, Clevers H. Tracking adult stem cells. EMBO Rep 2011;12(2) 113-22.

[100] Levy V, Lindon C, Harfe BD, Morgan BA. Distinct stem cell populations regenerate the follicle and interfollicular epidermis. Dev Cell 2005;9(6) 855-61.

[101] Sommer L. Checkpoints of melanocyte stem cell development. Sci STKE 2005;2005(298) pe42.

[102] Gir P, Oni G, Brown SA, Mojallal A, Rohrich RJ. Human adipose stem cells: current clinical applications. Plast Reconstr Surg 2012;129(6) 1277-90.

[103] Martin U. Methods for studying stem cells: adult stem cells for lung repair. Methods 2008;45(2) 121-32.

[104] Roche R, Hoareau L, Mounet F, Festy F. Adult stem cells for cardiovascular diseases: the adipose tissue potential. Expert Opin Biol Ther 2007;7(6) 791-8.

[105] Takahashi K, Yamanaka S. Induction of pluripotent stem cells from mouse embryonic and adult fibroblast cultures by defined factors. Cell 2006;126(4) 663-76.

[106] Chin MH, Mason MJ, Xie W, Volinia S, Singer M, Peterson C, et al. Induced pluripotent stem cells and embryonic stem cells are distinguished by gene expression signatures. Cell Stem Cell 2009;5(1) 111-23.

[107] Guenther MG, Frampton GM, Soldner F, Hockemeyer D, Mitalipova M, Jaenisch R, et al. Chromatin structure and gene expression programs of human embryonic and induced pluripotent stem cells. Cell Stem Cell 2010;7(2) 249-57.

[108] Newman AM, Cooper JB. Lab-specific gene expression signatures in pluripotent stem cells. Cell Stem Cell 2010;7(2) 258-62.

[109] Doi A, Park IH, Wen B, Murakami P, Aryee MJ, Irizarry R, et al. Differential methylation of tissue- and cancer-specific CpG island shores distinguishes human induced pluripotent stem cells, embryonic stem cells and fibroblasts. Nat Genet 2009;41(12) 1350-3.

[110] Boland MJ, Hazen JL, Nazor KL, Rodriguez AR, Gifford W, Martin G, et al. Adult mice generated from induced pluripotent stem cells. Nature 2009;461(7260) 91-4.

[111] Raya A, Rodriguez-Piza I, Guenechea G, Vassena R, Navarro S, Barrero MJ, et al. Disease-corrected haematopoietic progenitors from Fanconi anaemia induced pluripotent stem cells. Nature 2009;460(7251) 53-9.

[112] Hanna J, Wernig M, Markoulaki S, Sun CW, Meissner A, Cassady JP, et al. Treatment of sickle cell anemia mouse model with iPS cells generated from autologous skin. Science 2007;318(5858) 1920-3.

[113] Friedl P, Wolf K. Tube travel: the role of proteases in individual and collective cancer cell invasion. Cancer Res 2008;68(18) 7247-9.

[114] Beningo KA, Dembo M, Wang YL. Responses of fibroblasts to anchorage of dorsal extracellular matrix receptors. Proc Natl Acad Sci U S A 2004;101(52) 18024-9.

[115] Kalluri R, Zeisberg M. Fibroblasts in cancer. Nat Rev Cancer 2006;6(5) 392-401.

[116] Singer CF, Gschwantler-Kaulich D, Fink-Retter A, Haas C, Hudelist G, Czerwenka K, et al. Differential gene expression profile in breast cancer-derived stromal fibroblasts. Breast Cancer Res Treat 2008;110(2) 273-81.

[117] Tuxhorn JA, Ayala GE, Rowley DR. Reactive stroma in prostate cancer progression. J Urol 2001;166(6) 2472-83.

[118] Sato M, Sato T, Kojima N, Imai K, Higashi N, Wang DR, et al. 3-D structure of extracellular matrix regulates gene expression in cultured hepatic stellate cells to induce process elongation. Comp Hepatol 2004;3 Suppl 1 S4.

[119] Paszek MJ, Zahir N, Johnson KR, Lakins JN, Rozenberg GI, Gefen A, et al. Tensional homeostasis and the malignant phenotype. Cancer Cell 2005;8(3) 241-54.

[120] Chua A, Song C, Chai A, Kong S, Tan KC. Use of skin allograft and its donation rate in Singapore: an 11-year retrospective review for burns treatment. Transplant Proc 2007;39(5) 1314-6.

[121] Goel A, Shrivastava P. Post-burn scars and scar contractures. Indian J Plast Surg 2010;43(Suppl) S63-71.

[122] Harrison CA, Gossiel F, Layton CM, Bullock AJ, Johnson T, Blumsohn A, et al. Use of an in vitro model of tissue-engineered skin to investigate the mechanism of skin graft contraction. Tissue Eng 2006;12(11) 3119-33.

[123] Meier F, Nesbit M, Hsu MY, Martin B, Van Belle P, Elder DE, et al. Human melanoma progression in skin reconstructs : biological significance of bFGF. Am J Pathol 2000;156(1) 193-200.

[124] Eves P, Layton C, Hedley S, Dawson RA, Wagner M, Morandini R, et al. Characterization of an in vitro model of human melanoma invasion based on reconstructed human skin. Br J Dermatol 2000;142(2) 210-22.

[125] Barker CL, McHale MT, Gillies AK, Waller J, Pearce DM, Osborne J, et al. The development and characterization of an in vitro model of psoriasis. J Invest Dermatol 2004;123(5) 892-901.

[126] Ferrari S, Pellegrini G, Matsui T, Mavilio F, De Luca M. Gene therapy in combination with tissue engineering to treat epidermolysis bullosa. Expert Opin Biol Ther 2006;6(4) 367-78.

[127] Petersen TH, Calle EA, Zhao L, Lee EJ, Gui L, Raredon MB, et al. Tissue-engineered lungs for in vivo implantation. Science;329(5991) 538-41.

[128] Macchiarini P, Jungebluth P, Go T, Asnaghi MA, Rees LE, Cogan TA, et al. Clinical transplantation of a tissue-engineered airway. Lancet 2008;372(9655) 2023-30.

[129] Jungebluth P, Alici E, Baiguera S, Le Blanc K, Blomberg P, Bozoky B, et al. Tracheobronchial transplantation with a stem-cell-seeded bioartificial nanocomposite: a proof-of-concept study. Lancet 2011;378(9808) 1997-2004.

Naturally Derived Biomaterials: Preparation and Application

Tran Le Bao Ha, To Minh Quan,
Doan Nguyen Vu and Do Minh Si

Additional information is available at the end of the chapter

1. Introduction

The success of any implant depends so much on the biomaterial used. Naturally derived biomaterials have been demonstrated to show several advantages compared to synthetic biomaterials. These are biocompatibility, biodegradability and remodeling. Therefore, these biomaterials are usually applied in the repair or replacement of damaged human tissues and organs. The aim of this chapter is to provide a brief knowledge of naturally derived biomaterials as well as methods of preparation and application of them.

Biomaterials can be classified into two main groups: synthetic and natural biomaterials. Synthetic biomaterials are classified as: metals, ceramics, nonbiodegradable polymers, biodegradable polymers... Some synthetic biomaterials are commercialized and applied in clinical treatment such as metal hip, Dacron, plastic intraocular lens... However, synthetic biomaterials have some disadvantages, including their structure and composition is not similar to native tissues/organs, their biocompatibility and their ability to induce tissue remodeling are low. Thus, other biomaterials have been developed that can overcome the disadvantages of synthetic biomaterials. Today, naturally derived biomaterials have been attracting scientist's interest all over the world. Naturally derived biomaterial can be classified into many groups including protein-based biomaterials (collagen, gelatin, silk...), polysaccharide-based biomaterials (cellulose, chitin/chitosan, glucose...) and decellularized tissue-derived biomaterials (decellularized heart valves, blood vessels, liver...). Protein and polysaccharide-based biomaterials can be prepared by two distinct ways. Protein and polysaccharide from living organisms are dissolved by solvents or enzymes. Then, they are precipitated and reconstituted into fibrils. The second way to prepare protein and polysaccharide is removing other elements of living organisms by solvents or enzymes. Decellularized biomaterials are created by eliminating all cells from native tissues/organs. Physical, chemical and enzymatic approaches are combined to make the effective decellularization protocol.

Because of their advantages, naturally derived biomaterials are usually applied to replace or restore structure and function of damaged tissues/organs. They have ability to adequately support cell adhesion, migration, proliferation and differentiation. In particular, when implanted into a defective area, naturally derived biomaterials can enhance the attachment and migration of cells from the surrounding environment, therefore, induce extracellular matrix formation and promote tissue repair. Some biomaterials are used to acting as drug delivery system and medical devices such as surgical sutures. The silk fiber produced by silkworm or spider has been used as a surgical suture for a long time due to its biodegradable and non-antigenic protein. These silk fibroin nanoparticles are the globules with a fine crystallinity that may offer various possibilities for surface modification and covalent drug attachment. Furthermore, some biomaterials are used to produce environmental friendliness of packaging (such as resorbable chitosan packing) and other products. Some commercial products were made from naturally derived biomaterial such as SIS, Matrigel, Alloderm... In this chapter, we focus on a brief knowledge as well as the methods of preparation and application of naturally derived biomaterials in our researches.

2. Naturally derived biomaterials: Preparation and application

2.1. Protein

2.1.1. Collagen

2.1.1.1. Structure

Collagen is the most abundant protein of connective tissues in all animals. Now, at least sixteen types of collagen have been identified, in which 80-90% of the collagen is types I, II and III. Collagen is secreted by not only fibroblasts but also epithelial cells [1].

The basic structural unit of collagen is a triple helix. Most collagen is fibrillar because of pack of collagen molecules type I, II, III. Contrast, collagen IV forms a two dimensional network which is unique to the basement membranes [1]. Basement membranes have been performed a number of mechanical and biological functions. They provide physical support for tissue because of their tensile strength. They also influence cell proliferation, adhesion, migration, differentiation, polarization, and are thus implicated in biological processes such as development, tissue maintenance, regeneration, and repair, and in various pathological processes such as tumor growth and metastasis [2].

The basement membranes composition varies from one tissue to another. In general, the major constituents of all basement membranes are collagen IV, laminins, nidogen/entactin, and proteoglycans. The functional diversity of basement membranes arises from the molecular diversity of their components, particularly the different collagen IV and laminin isoforms [2].

2.1.1.2. Preparation

Collagen can be obtained from various sources, in which amniotic membrane (AM) is an attractive source. AM is a thin membrane surrounding the fetus which is filled with amniotic fluid.

The AM consists of an epithelial monolayer, a thick basement membrane, a compact layer, a fibroblast layer and a spongy layer [3]. The innermost layer, nearest to the fetus, is monolayer of epithelial cells anchored on the basement membrane. The collagen component of basement membrane of AM includes types III, IV, V, VII, XVII which similar morphological and ultra-structural basement membrane of skin. Therefore, basement membrane of AM is often used to create skin equivalents. Besides, AM has outstanding properties such as anti-inflammatory, anti-bacterial, anti-fibrosis, anti-scaring as well as low immunogenicity and reasonable mechanical features [3].

AM can be used either with amniotic epithelium (intact) or without it (denuded), fresh or preserved. To remove the amniotic epithelium, the AM is incubated in trypsin-EDTA at 37°C in 30 min and the cells are gently scraped while maintaining the intact basement membrane. H&E staining was performed to confirm removing the amniotic epithelium. Then, the basement membrane can be preserved by drying or glycerol - cryopreservation after γ-sterilization [3, 4, 5].

2.1.1.3. Application

Collagen is commonly used in biomedical applications. The basement membrane of the AM is a typical example. The extracellular matrix components of the basement membrane of the AM are native scaffolds for cell seeding in tissue engineering. AM has been applied in tissue engineering related to eye, skin, cartilage, nerve, especially cancer [3, 6, 7].

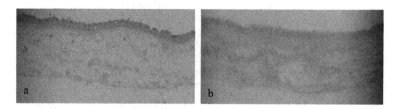

Figure 1. Amniotic membrane with epithelium: intact (a) and denuded (b)

To use AM in creating skin equivalent, AM must be removed the epithelium. Keratinocytes are seeded onto basement membrane which is denuded AM. Briefly, keratinocytes were iso-lated from intact skin samples by incubation in trypsin-EDTA at 4°C in 18 hours and detach-ed mechanically. Keratinocytes were cultured in serum free medium in 7 days. Medium was chanced every two days [8]. After 3rd passage, cells were subcultured onto AM basement membrane which spreaded on bottom of the insert dishes. The cells were maintained in cul-ture for 7 days when the cells reached confluent. Air-lifting was performed to induce cell differentiation. After 7 days, the cells formed multi-layers on the AM basement membrane. Cultured keratinocyte sheets were grafted on patients who were defected skin because of injury or burn. The result showed that, the advantages of cultured keratinocyte sheet autograft: the possibility of the grafting area multiplication (50 times after 3 weeks), the diminution of scaring, the relief of pain, the low infection risk, the same effect in compare to the split - thinness autograft.

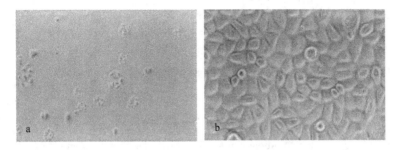

Figure 2. Keratinocytes formed colonies (a) and monolayer onto culture dishes (b) (200X)

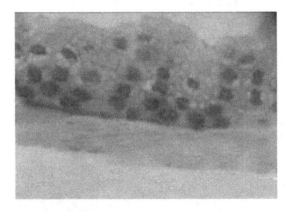

Figure 3. Result of HE staining of the cell sheet, the cells were exposed to the air in seven days. The cells formed 4 – 5 layers onto AM basement membrane (400X).

2.2. Gelatin-Alginate

2.2.1. Structure

Gelatin is obtained by controlling the hydrolysis of collagen, a fibrous insoluble protein which is widely found in nature and is the major component of skin, bone and connective tissue. Characteristic features of gelatin are the high content of the amino acids such as glycine, proline and hydroxyproline. Structually, gelatin molecules contain repeating sequences of glycine-X-Y triplets, where X and Y are frequently proline and hydroxyproline. These sequences are responsible for the triple helical structure of gelatin and its ability to form gels where helical regions form in the gelatin protein chains immobilizing water [9].

Alginate was first discovered by Edward Stanford in 1883. Since being commercialized in 1927, alginate has now expanded to about 50.000 tonnes per year worldwide; 30% of this tonnage is devoted to the food industry, the rest being used in industrial, pharmaceutical and dental applications [10]. The function of alginates in algae is primarily skeletal, with the gel located in the cell wall and intercellular matrix conferring the strength and flexibility necessary to withstand the force of water in which the seaweed grows [11].

Alginate is a hydrophilic polysaccharide extracted from marine brown algae such as Laminaria hyperborea or soil bacteria such as Azobacter vinelandii and composed of 1,4-linked β-D-mannuronic acid (M) residues and 1,4-linked α-L-guluronic acid (G) in varying proportions, displaying carboxylic acid functionality at the C5 residue. The alginates have broad distributions of molecular weights of 10-1000 kDa depending on source and processing. The relative amount and sequential distribution of homogeneous M-M segments (M-blocks), homogeneous G-G segments (G-blocks) and alternating M-G segments (MG-blocks), which represent the primary structure of alginate, depend on the producing species, and for marine sources, on seasonal and geographical variations.

2.2.2. Preparation

Cross-linked gelatin/alginate was made in two steps. Briefly, 1wt % (w/w) aqueous solution of gelatin and sodium alginate, respectively, was dissolved in double distilled water at 500C for 3 h. Each solution with certain mixing ratios of gelatin and sodium alginate (8G:2A) was stirred for 30min at room temperature, frozen to -700C for 40 h. This soluble sponge was cross-linked with EDC by immersing the soluble sponge in 90% (w/v) aqueous acetone containing 0.3% EDC for 24 h at room temperature, while shaking slowly.

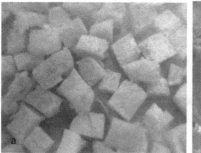 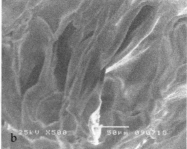

Figure 4. Gelatin-Alginate. Block (a), SEM (b)

The sponges consisting of gelatin from hydrolysis of collagen and alginate-a polysaccharide from Phaeophyta were established by using EDC as a crosslinking agent. The sponges were combined with some natural substances traditional used for burn treatment such as tamanu oil (from nuts of Calophyllum inophyllum); cajeputi oil (from leaves of Meulaleuca leucadendron); madecassol (from extract of Centella asiatica); turmeric and python fat. Data obtained from testing on mice showed that the coordinated sponges have rather good ability on preventing infection and promoting wound healing compared with control. The sponges combined with mixture of cajeputi oil and madecassol have the best potential for burn treatment.

2.2.3. Application

Gelatin has been used in medicine as plasma expander, wound dressing, adhesive, and absorbent pad for surgical use. While collagen, also known to have wide biomedical applications, expresses antigenicity in physiological condition, gelatin is known to have no such antigenicity. Recently, gelatin has shown to exhibit activation of macrophages and high hemostatic effect. Finally, gelatin is practically more convenient than collagen because a concentrated collagen solution is extremely difficult to prepare from the native collagen, and furthermore gelatin is far more economical than the collagen.

Alginate is an effective natural disintegrant, tablet binder and offers an attractive alternative for sustained-release systems. It offers advantages over synthetic polymers as it forms hydrogels under relatively mild pH and temperature and is generally regarded as non-toxic, biocompatible, biodegradable, less expensive and abundantly available in nature; in addition, alginate meets the important requirement of being amenable to sterilization and storage. All these advantages make alginates very useful materials for biomedical applications, especially for controlled delivery of drugs and other biologically active compounds and for the encapsulation of cells. Calcium alginate is a natural haemostat, so alginate based dressings are indicated for bleeding wounds. The gel forming property of alginate helps in removing the dressing without much trauma [12].

Alginate has been much used in medical applications such as wound dressings, scaffolds for hepatocyte culture and surgical or dental impression materials. Alginates are also known to be broken down to simpler glucose type residues and can be totally absorbed.

Alginate has been successfully used as a matrix for the entrapment and/or delivery of biological agents, such as drugs and proteins. In particular proteins can be loaded and released by alginate matrices without loss of their biological activity because of the relatively mild gelation process of alginate. In pharmaceutical formulations, the alginate gel can be prepared prior to use, or it can spontaneously form in situ in physiological fluids, by low pH and/or calcium ions naturally present in the site of administration [13]. Alternatively, the gelling agent can be added either as a part of the formulation or separately administered. The microencapsulation technique has been specifically developed for the oral delivery of proteins, as they are quickly denatured and degraded in the hostile environment of the stomach.

Among the possible applications of alginate, one of the most promising is for cell immobilization. Alginate gel allows cell suspension to be cultivated in several types of bioreactors to achieve high cell densities [14]. In cell immobilization applications, the main drawback of alginate matrix gels is represented by their high density of network, which limits the cell growth; moreover, cell anchorage, a strict requirement for survival, is limited on alginate gels, because of its hydrophilic nature. PEG copolymers are used to improve their biocompatibility [15].

2.3. Silk

Silks are generally defined as protein polymers that are spun into fibers by Lepidoptera larvae such as silkworms, spiders, scorpions, mites and flies [16]. Silks are fibrous proteins synthesized in specialized epithelial cells that line glands in these organisms. Silk fibroin polymers consist of repetitive protein sequences and provide structural roles in cocoon formation, nest building, traps, web formation, safety lines and egg protection. The most extensively used silk for various applications are those from silkworm silk; Bombyx mori and spider silk; Nephila clavipes.

The domesticated silkworm (B. mori) silk fibroin fibers are about 10–25 μm in diameter. Each fiber consists of core protein covered by a coating protein (sericin) that glues core fibers together. The core protein consists of three chains: heavy chain, light chain and a glycoprotein, P25. The light chain (26 kDa) and heavy chain (390 kDa) which are present in a 1:1 ratio and linked by a single disulfide bond. The disulfide linkage between the Cys-c20 (20th residue from the carboxyl terminus) of the heavy chain and Cys-172 of the light chain holds the fibroin together and a 25 kDa glycoprotein, named P25, is non-covalently linked to these proteins [17]. Light chain is necessary for the secretion of protein from the silk glands. Heavy chain is fiber forming protein and its structure determines properties of silk fiber [18]. Heavy chain is commonly referred as fibroin protein. These proteins are coated with a family of hydrophilic proteins called sericins (20–310 kDa). Silk proteins are particularly promising for these needs due to their unique combination of biocompatibility, biodegradability, self-assembly, mechanical stability, controllable structure and morphology.

Spiders are look like insects and come in to the category of Arthropoda, but they belong to a completely different class of animals, called Arachnida. Spider silk is the result of 400 million years of evolution. Spiders use silk for variety of functions including reproduction as cocoon capsular structures, lines for prey capture, lifeline support (dragline), web construction and adhesion. Spider silk is a biopolymer fiber. Its composition is a mix of an amorphous polymer (which makes the fiber elastic), and chains of two of the simplest proteins (which give it toughness). Out of 20 amino acids, only Glycine and Alanine serve as a primary constituent of silk. The Dragline silk of orbweb spider seems to be most studied in the scientific research. The protein in dragline silk is fibroin (Mass of 200,000-300,000 Daltons) which is a combination of the proteins spidroin 1 (Alanine-rich) and spidroin 2 (Glycine-rich), the exact composition of these proteins depends on species. Fibroin consists of approximately 40% Glycine and 25% Alanine as the major amino acids. The remaining components are mostly glutamine, serine, leucine, valine, proline, tyrosine and arginine [19]. Nephila clavipes can produce seven types of silk from seven different silk glands as shown in depending on needs and environmental conditions [20]. The superior mechanical properties of dragline spider silks can be used as a template for developing specific structures for various biomaterial needs. Spider silks have not been commercialized in fashion as silkworm silk due to the lack of domestication and lower productivity of spiders.

2.3.1. Preparation

Nanotechnology is becoming a key technology and capable of application in all fields of science and technology. In particular, nanoparticle delivery system significantly improved pharmaceutical treatment of many incurable diseases which require complex treatment regimens, as well as, patients must take multiple medications and need time long-term drug use. Silk Protein is the ideal material for this purpose, because they have many unique features such as highly biocompatible and biodegradable ability, self-restructuring, mechanical stability, easy control and adjustment of the object's structure and shape.

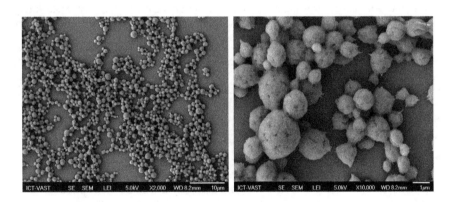

Figure 5. Nanofibroin particles

The cocoon shell of silkworm Bombyx mori was degummed in boiling solution of 0,5% Na2CO3 in 700C for 35 min. Then degummed fiber was dissolved in a mixed solution of calcium chloride, ethanol, and water (CaCl2/C2H5OH/H2O: 1:2:8 mole ratio), at 800C. After the silk fibroin–salts solution was centrifuged at 5000 rpm for 10 min, the supernatant was dialyzed continuously for 72 h against running pure water to remove CaCl2, smaller molecules, and some impurities. The resulting liquid silk fibroin was stored at 40C and used in the following experiments for the preparation of silk fibroin nanoparticles. Spider silk proteins form nanoparticles upon salting out with potassium phosphate. Milk-like silk protein particles were formed at once and suspended in the mixture comprising water and organic solvent. These protein particles were water insoluble and went down slowly due to the gathering of microparticles. The precipitates of silk protein nanoparticles were collected and purified from the mixture by repeated centrifugation at 20,000 rpm to separate these particles from the solvent. After the research, we have obtained nanoparticles (500 nm-2000 nm) from silk protein can load and delivery of proteins in vitro.

2.3.2. Application

The silk bio-polymer is used in tissue regeneration for treating burn victims and as matrix of wound healing. The silk fibroin peptides are used in cosmetics due to their glossy, flexible, elastic coating power, easy spreading and adhesion characters [21]. Silk powder is touted and relieves from sunburns, due to crystalline structure it reflects UV radiation and as demulcent it acts as protective buffer between skin and environment. The lower micron silk powder is added with hair and massage oils and water dispersible finer grade silk powder is an ingredient of liquid cosmetic preparations.

The silk is used to fight edema, cystitis, impotence, adenosine augmentation therapy, epididymitis and cancer [22]. Silk protein derivative, Serratio peptidase is used as anti-inflammatory, anti-tumefacient for treating acute sinusitis, tonsiloctomy, oral surgery, tooth filling, cleaning and extractions. The silk fibroin is a useful dressing material with the property of non-cytotoxic to the tissues and also in veterinary medication.

Since long, silk fiber is being used as surgical sutures as it does not cause inflammatory reactions and is absorbed after wounds heal. Other promising medical applications are as biodegradable micro tubes for repair of blood vessels and as molded inserts for bone, cartilage and teeth reconstruction [23, 24, 25]. In biomedical and bioengineered field, the use of natural fibre mixed with biodegradable and bio-resorbable polymers can produce joints and bone fixtures to alleviate pain for patients.

Drug delivery is a rapidly developing field in biomedical research. It is interdisciplinary and requires expertise in biotechnology, pharmacology, microbiology, biochemistry, polymer chemistry and materials engineering. Advantages of using such systems include maintenance of drug levels within desired range, fewer administrations, optimal use of the drug, and better patient compliance. The material used for drug delivery should be biocompatible, chemically inert, easily processable and physically and mechanically stable. Biopolymers are of great interest for this kind of application. Silk and silk-like variants are used by some scientists as carriers for drug delivery. Their biocompatibility and ability to form hydrogels in situ makes them attractive candidates for the localized, controlled delivery of therapeutic agents. Their ability to incorporate drugs at room temperature, by simple mixing, and without the use of toxic or denaturing solvents makes them attractive for the delivery of protein or DNA-based therapies [26].

Future applications of silk biomaterials include new generation soft contact lenses that enable greater oxygen permeability, artificial corneas, skin grafts and epilepsy drug permeable devices.

2.4. Fibrin

2.4.1. Structure

The mechanism of fibrin fomation is elucidated primarily from the thrombin-mediated cleavage of fibrinogen. Fibrinogen, the principal protein of blood clotting, is a 340 kDa trinolar protein which presents at high concentration in blood plasma (2 – 4 mg/ml, 6 – 12 μM). Fibrinogen molecule consists of three different pairs of polypeptide chains (Aα, Bβ and γ) cross-linked to each other by 29 disulfide bridges (Fig. 1). The amine-termini (N-termini) of six polypeptide chains are converged in the central of fibrinogen molecule called the E domain. The carboxy-termini (C-termini) of the Bβ chain and γ chain comprise of the distal D domain. The C-termini of Aα chains which are known as globular, depart from the D domain and fold into a conformation that stretches back toward the E domain of fibrinogen [27].

Fibrinogen plays as precursor protein of fibrin in blood clotting. The conversion of fibrinogen to fibrin occurs in 3 ordered steps. In the intinial step, thrombin binds to the central E domain of fibrinogen and slipts off the fibrinopeptides A – FpA (16 amino acid residues) and B – FpB (14 amino acid residues) from N-termini of Aα and Bβ chains, respectively, whereas the γ chains remain unaltered. The cleavage of FpA and FpB results in exposure of "A" and "B" binding sites. Then, the self-assembly proccess will spontaneously occur. The "A" and "B" sites will interact with complementary sites ("a" and "b" sites located in the γ and β chain) at the D domain of other fibrinogen molecules, which results in new fibrin monomers. The fibrin monomers are bound to each other non-covalently (Fig. 2) and assemble in a half-staggered manner into two-stranded protofibrils which continue to aggregate laterally to form fibers branching into a three-dimensional network of fibrin [28, 29]. Finally, fibrin cross-linking is activated by Factor XIII (FXIII) in order to improve the strong and elastic properties, additionally, avoid fibrinolysis in solution [30, 31].

2.4.2. Fabrication of fibrin gel

According to the usage purposes, some methods have been applied to fabricate fibrin gels. Fibrin gels can be conducted either from the separating components including thrombin, fibrinogen and CaCl2, or from serum of patients, which will be mentioned in two following methods, respectively. For manipulation of fibrin gel from separating commercial components, fibrin gels were prepared by combining fibrinogen, NaCl, thrombin, CaCl2. This complex is also supplemented with aprotinin in order to proving a stable fibrin structure and prevents postoperative bleeding. The contents are allowed to gel for 1 hr in standard culture conditions [32]. Furthermore, fibrin gel physical properties can be manipulated by adjusting the fibrinogen and $CaCl_2$ concentration [33, 34], or using different cross linking agents such as enzymes or UV radiation [35]. In terms of autologous fibrin glue, the patient blood is havested and prepared 3 to 4 days before surgery. The plasma is separated from red blood cells by allowing the blood tube to stand vertically for at least 2 hours or centrifuged at 4000 rmp for 5 minutes. The fibrin gel preparation is created by combining plasma with commercial thrombin and calcium at appropriate concentration [36]. Autologous plasma fibrin gel not only shows an excellent hemostatic agent, but also helps eliminate the risk of viral transmission associated using donor plasma.

2.4.3. Fibrin gel applications

Numerous studies have exploited fibrin function as heamostatic plug, scaffold for cell proliferation and migration, and wound healing, which suggest fibrin potential applications in medical and tissue engineering. Fibrin glue or fibrin sealant is a formulation of fibrinogen and thrombin at very high amounts cobined with calcium and FXIII, used as an adjunct to hemostasis in patients undergoing surgery. Commercial products of fibrin sealant such as Tisseel (Immuno, Vienna, Austria), Beriplast (Behringwerke AG, Marburg/Lahn, FRG), and Biocol (CRTS, Lille, France) have been extensively used in clinical. In addition to fibrin'role in heamostatic, fibrin is also indicated as biological scaffold for cell proliferation, migration and differentiation applied in various tissue engineering. Natural fibrin matrix consists of sites for cellular binding, and has been shown to have excellent effects in cell culture and accelabrate tissue regeneration. In 2000, Ye et al. fabricated and investigated the three-dimensional fibrin scaffold in cardiovascular tissue engineering. In this research, human myofibroblasts (MFBs) from the ascending aorta were cultured in fibrin gel solution. Consequently, the cell growth, high collagen secretation and tissue development were determined. Besides, toxic degradation or inflammatory reactions was not detected in the fibrin gels [37]. In 2003, W. Bensa.id and colleagues conducted a research in which they use fibrin glue as a delivery system for human MSCs (HMSCs). The result confirmed a good good HMSCs spreading and proliferation in the fibrin scaffold. Besides, the HMSCs migration out of the fibrin scaffold and appearance of calcium carbonate from the differentiation of HMSCs when implanted in vivo suggest that fibrin gel is a promising delivery system for HMSCs toward bone healing application [38]. Fibrin glue also performs its role in the application of skin grafts to burned areas. Using fibrin glue instead of sutures or pressure dressings in the immediate postoperative period enhances healing, and minimizes scarring [39]. One of commercial fibrin sealant products used for burn treatment is ARTISS fibrin sealant (Baxter International Inc., USA). ARTISS fibrin sealant is indicated to adhere autologous skin grafts to surgically prepared wound beds resulting from burns, for both adults and pedipatients.

3. Polysaccharide

3.1. Cellulose

3.1.1. Structure

Cellulose is the most abundant polymer on Earth, which makes it also the most common organic compound. Annual cellulose synthesis by plants is close to 10^{12} tons. Plants contain approximately 33% cellulose whereas wood contains around 50% and cotton contains 90%. Most of the cellulose is utilised as a raw material in paper production. This equates to approximately 10^8 tons of pulp produced annually. From this, only 4 million tons are used for further chemical processing annually. It is quite clear from these values that only a very small fraction of cellulose is used for the production of commodity materials and chemicals [40]. Cellulose, a linear polysaccharide of up to 15,000 D-glucose residues linked by β-(1→4)-glycosidic bonds, is biocompatible and has excellent thermal, mechanical properties. It is considered easily biodegradable, thus less contaminating to the environment.

Cellulose is regarded as a semi-flexible polymer. The relative stiffness and rigidity of the cellulose molecule is mainly due to the intramolecular hydrogen bonding. This property is reflected in its high viscosity in solution, a high tendency to crystallise, and its ability to form fibrillar strands. The chain stiffness property is further favoured by the β-glucosidic linkage that bestows the linear form of the chain. The chair conformation of the pyranose ring also contributes to chain stiffness. This is in contrast to the α-glucosidic bonds of starch [41].

Plants are an attractive cellulose source primarily because they are abundant and there is a preexisting infrastructure in the textile industries for harvesting, retting/pulping (i.e. to treat and isolate micron sized cellulose particles), and product processing. Tunicates are the only animals known to produce cellulose microfibrils. Tunicates are a family of sea animals that have a mantle consisting of cellulose microfibrils embedded in a protein matrix. It is this thick leathery mantle in their mature phase that is used as a source of cellulose microfibrils. Most research has used a class of Tunicates that are commonly known as "sea squirts" (*Ascidiacea*), marine invertebrate filter feeders. Several algae species such as green, gray, red, yellow-green… produce cellulose microfibrils in the cell wall. There are considerable differences in cellulose microfibril structure between the various algae species caused by differences in the biosynthesis process. Most cellulose microfibril researchers have used various species of green algae. Bacterial cellulose (BC) is a glucose polymer produced through bacterial fermentation. This macromolecular polymer features the same molecular formula and properties of natural cellulose. A fiber bundle of 40 to 60 nm thick is formed by micro-fibers with a diameter range of 3 to 4 nm. These bundles aggregate randomly to produce a developed structure forming a typical type of nanobiomaterial [42].

Cellulose derivatives and composites offer an excellent biocompatibility, and are considered as promising materials for biochemical engineering for economic and scientific reasons.

- Oxidized cellulose (oxycellulose) is cellulose in which some of the terminal primary alcohol groups of the glucose residues have been converted to carboxyl groups. Therefore, the product is possibly a synthetic polyanhydrocellobiuronide and that contain 25% carboxyl groups are too brittle and too readily soluble to be of use. Those products that have lower carboxyl contents are the most desirable[43].

- Purified microcrystalline cellulose (MCC) is partially depolymerized cellulose prepared by treating α-cellulose, obtained as a pulp from fibrous plant material, with mineral acids. Silicified MCC (SMCC) is manufactured by codrying a suspension of MCC particles and colloidal silicon dioxide such that the dried finished product contains 2% colloidal silicon dioxide. SMCC shows higher bulk density than the common types of MCC. Also, tensile strength of compacts of SMCC is greater than that of the respective MCC and it is most probably a consequence of intersurface interactions of silicon dioxide and MCC [44]

- The esterification can be considered as a typical equilibrium reaction in which an alcohol and acid react to form ester and water. Cellulose is esterified with certain acids such as acetic acid, nitric acid, sulfuric acid, and phosphoric acid. A prerequisite is that the acid used can bring about a strong swelling thus penetrating throughout the cellulose structure. Cellulose acetate phthalate is a partial acetate ester of cellulose that has been reacted with phthalic anhydride. One carboxyl of the phthalic acid is esterified with the cellulose acetate. The finished product contains about 20% acetyl groups and about 35% phthalyl groups [45].

3.1.2. Preparation

The treatments for wood and plants involve the complete or partial removal of matrix materials (hemicellulose, lignin, etc.) and the isolation of individual complete fibers. Fortunicate the treatment involves the isolation of the mantel from the animal and the isolation of individual cellulose fibrils with the removal of the protein matrix. Treatments for algal cellulose sources typically involve culturing methods, and then purifying steps for removal of algal wall matrix material. Bacterial cellulose treatments focus on culturing methods for cellulose microfibrillar growth and then washing to remove the bacteria and other media.

The general processing of engineered BC materials can be considered to occur in four main stages: (1) BC culturing, (2) pellicle management, (3) water removal, and (4) chemical modification. For stage 1, the biosynthesis of BC occurs in culture solutions, generally in a bioreactor, in which bacteria secrete cellulose microfibrils, producing an interwoven web of fibrils that is a hydrogel. The hydrogels are composed of entangled cellulose microfibrils formed from the random motion of the bacteria, contain upwards of 99% water, and are called pellicles. For stage 2, pellicle management refers to any process imparted on the pellicle up until the point of water removal. To remove the bacteria from the pellicles, the pellicles are washed by boiling in a low concentration (2%) NaOH bath for several hours, then it is rinsed under running water for several days. Additional NaOH and NaClO treatments have also been used for further purification of the BC microfibrils. For stage 3, once the pellicle is formed and purified, a sample is cut from the gel-like sheet. Water removal either by evaporation or a combination of pressing and evaporation collapses the gel-network and produces a dense film. For stage 4, chemical modification to the BC microfibril network can be achieved at three points along the engineered BC material processing, (i) during stage 1, (ii) during stage 2, and (iii) after stage 3 (i.e. to dried BC structures or films) [42].

3.1.3. Application

Cellulose is extensively used as a raw material in the paper industry in the production of paper and cardboard products. However, cellulose has shown its versatility in numerous applications.

Natural cellulose spheres are often applied in bioseparation, immobilized reaction, cell suspension culture, and as an adsorbent for sewage treatment. Spherical BC produced from dynamic method is translucent, loose, porous, and has a hydrophilic network structure. Its specific surface area increases with decreasing spherical diameter, so it could be used as a carrier to adsorb or crosslink various kinds of substances (e.g., enzyme, cell, protein, nucleic acid, and other compounds). Spherical BC may be applied in bioseparation, immobilized reaction, cell suspension culture, and as an adsorbent for sewage treatment. Compared with natural spherical cellulose, the fermentation production of BC spheres is simple, controllable and environment friendly. Moreover, BC sphere can be used repeatedly, expanding their potential applications.

Cellulosic derivatives such as cellulose acetate, cellulose propionate and cellulose acetate-butyrate, cast as membranes, have been reported as useful supports for immobilizing various enzymes such as catalase, alcohol oxidase and glucose oxidase. These supports gave better activity and storage stability for the enzymes. Cellulose ethers are widely used as important excipients for designing matrix tablets. On contact with water, the cellulose ethers start to swell and the hydrogel layer starts to grow around the dry core of the tablet. The hydrogel presents a diffusional barrier for water molecules penetrating into the polymer matrix and the drug molecules being released. Cellulose acetate butyrate microcapsules, as well as cellulose-based microspheres, have been used for the delivery of drugs [46].

Microbial cellulose synthesized by *Acetobacter xylinum* shows considerable potential as a novel wound healing system, resulting from its unique nanostructure. During the process of biosynthesis, various carbon compounds of the nutrition medium are utilized by the bacteria, then polymerized into single, linear β-1,4-glucan chains and finally secreted outside the cells through a linear row of pores located on their outer membrane. Cellulose derived from *Acetobacter xylinum*, as discussed above in the context of wound healing, has also been explored as a potential scaffold material, due to its unusual material properties and degradability. Moreover, bacterial cellulose derived from *Acetobacter xylinum* has an ultrafine network architecture, high hydrophilicity, and mouldability during formation. In addition to the applications discussed, it is also suitable for use in micronerve surgery and as an artificial blood vessel suitable for microsurgery [47].

3.2. Chitin-Chitosan

3.2.1. Structure

Chitin is a white, hard, inelastic, nitrogenous polysaccharide found in the exoskeleton as well as in the internal structure of invertebrates. Chitin is a hydrophobic linear polysaccharide derived from many natural sources including the exoskeleton of arthropods and insects and is the second most abundant natural polysaccharide next to cellulose. Chitin comprises a polysaccharide consisting of $(1\rightarrow4)$-β-N-acetyl-D-glucosamine units. Derivatives of chitin may be classified into two categories; in each case, the N-acetyl groups are removed, and the exposed amino function then reacts either with acyl chlorides or anhydrides to give the group NHCOR or is modified by reductive amination to $NHCH_2COOH$ of greatest potential importance are derivatives of both types formed by reaction with bi or polyfunctional reagents, thus carrying sites for further chemical reaction [48]. In practice, such reactions are carried out on native chitin or on incompletely deacetylated chitin, chitosan, so that the resulting polymer contains three types of monomeric units.

Chitosan is a partially deacetylated derivative of chitin and is the second most abundant biosynthesized material. Structurally, chitosan is a mixture of N-acetyl-D-glucosamine and D-glucosamine [49]. Generally, chitosan is insoluble in neutral or basic conditions, while protonation of free amino groups facilitates solubility of chitosan in dilute acids (pH < 6). In vivo degradation of chitosan is mainly attributed to the effect of lysozyme through hydrolysis of acetylated residues.

Chitosan itself chelates metal ions, especially those of transition metals, and also finds application as a matrix for immobilization of enzymes. Special attention has been given to the chemical modification of chitin, since it has the greatest potential to be fully exploited. Reactions with pure chitin have been carried out mostly in the solid state owing to the lack of solubility in ordinary solvents. A 50% deacetylated chitin has been found to be soluble in water [50]. This water soluble form of chitin is a useful starting material for its smooth modifications, through various reactions in solution phase. Some of the very recently reported chitosan derivatives are enumerated as follows:

- Fully deacetylated chitosan was treated with phthalic anhydride to give N-phthaloyl-chitosan. It was readily soluble in polar organic solvents. Further reactions had been carried out using this new derivative to improve the solubility of chitosan [51].

- To improve water solubility, Sashiwa et al. has successfully synthesized dendronized chitosan-sialic acid hybrids by using gallic acid as focal point and tri(ethylene glycol) as spacer arm. The water solubility of these novel derivatives was further improved by N-succinylation of the remaining amine functionality [52].

- Recently, Baba et al. have synthesized methylthiocarbamoyl and phenylthiocarbamoyl chitosan derivatives to examine the selectivity toward metal ions from aqueous ammonium nitrate solution [53].

- The synthesis of chitosan hydrogels was carried out by Qu et al. by direct grafting of D,L-lactic and/or glycolic acid onto chitosan in the absence of catalysts. They demonstrated that a stronger interaction existed between water and chitosan chains after grafting lactic and/or glycolic acid. The side chains could aggregate and form physical crosslinking, which results in pH sensitive chitosan hydrogels [54].

3.2.2. Preparation

Chitin is easily obtained from crab or shrimp shells and fungal. In the first case, chitin production is associated with food industries such as shrimp canning. In the second case, the production of chitosan–glucan complexes is associated with fermentation processes, similar to those for the production of citric acid from *Aspergillus niger*, *Mucor rouxii*, and *Streptomyces*, which involves alkali treatment yielding chitosan–glucan complexes. The alkali removes the protein and deacetylates chitin simultaneously. Depending on the alkali concentration, some soluble glycans are removed. The processing of crustacean shells mainly involves the removal of proteins and the dissolution of calcium carbonate which is present in crab shells in high concentrations. The resulting chitin is deacetylated in 40% sodium hydroxide at 120^{0}C for 1–3 h. This treatment produces 70% deacetylated chitosan [55].

3.2.3. Application

Chitin and chitosan are known for their excellent biological properties, among which the biocompatibility with human cells, the ordered regeneration of wounded tissues, the immunoenhancing activity, the induction of immediate hemostasis, the radical scavenging activity, and the antimicrobial activity. Recent studies indicate that chitin and chitosan are most versatile in drug and gene delivery, elaborated diagnostics, devices for selective recognition of tumor cells, and surgical aids ranging from anti-adhesion gels to coated sterile stents.

As a kind of renewable resource, unmodified chitosan has been widely used in many fields such as pharmaceutical, agriculture, food, and biomedical applications. In order to realize the full potential of chitosan and bring a breakthrough in its broader utilization, attempts have been made to modify chitosan to obtain various derivatives. For the tissue repair and regeneration applications, chitosan can be functionalized by chemical reaction, coupling with specific ligands or moieties, combining with biomacromolecules, and crosslinking in the presence or absence of crosslinkers.

Particularly, skin substitute made of chitosan or its derivatives have attracted much attention due to the outstanding characteristics of chitosan, such as biocompatibility, hemostatic activity, antibacterial property, and ability to accelerate the wound-healing process [56].

The design of artificial kidney systems has made possible repetitive hemodialysis and the sustaining life of chronic kidney failure patients. Chitosan membranes have been proposed as an artificial kidney membrane because of their suitable permeability and high tensile strength. The most important part of artificial kidney is the semipermeable membrane and so far made from commercial regenerated cellulose and cuprophane. Since the primary action of the cellulose membrane is that of a sieve, there is little selectivity in the separation of two closely related molecules. These novel membranes need to be developed for better control of transport, ease of formability and inherent blood compatibility.

A series of membranes prepared from chitin and its derivatives improved dialysis properties. One of the most serious problems of using these artificial membranes is surface induced thrombosis, where heparization of blood is needed to prevent clotting, and people who are liable to internal hemorrhage can be dialysed only at great risk. Hence, these are the most challenging problem still to be resolved in the development of membranes which are inherently blood compatible. From these point of views, chitosan is hemostatic, i.e., causes clots [57].

Chitosan has replaced the synthetic polymers in opthalmological applications. Chitosan possesses all the characteristics required for an ideal contact lens; optical clarity, mechanical stability, sufficient optical correction, gas permeability, partially towards oxygen, wettability, and immunologically compatibility. Contact lenses are made from partially depolymerized and purified squid pen chitosan by spin casting technology, and these contact lenses are clear, tough, and possess other required physical properties such as modulus, tensile strength, tear strength, elongation, water content, and oxygen permeability. Antimicrobial and wound healing properties of chitosan along with excellent film forming capability make chitosan suitable for development of ocular bandage lens [58].

The special attention on chitosan has been paid for the repair of articular cartilage. Articular cartilage is particularly vulnerable to injury trama, disease or congenital abnormalities because of its avascular, alypmhatic and aneural nature. Once damaged, it has little capacity for intrinsic repair. Although many repair techniques have been attempted over the past four decades, but none has succeeded to regenerate long-lasting hyaline cartilage tissue to replace defected or damaged cartilage. Recently, preliminary studies on chitosan-GAG composite and its biologically interaction with articular chondrocytes showed promising results. Chitosan and its derivatives are being extensively used for bone tissue engineering and central nervous system also.

The growth of *Escherichia coli* was inhibited in the presence of chitosan. Chitosan also inhibited the growth of *Fusarium*, *Alternaria* and *Helminthosporium*. The cationic amino groups of chitosan probably bind to anionic groups of these microorganisms, resulting in growth inhibition. Extracellular lysozyme activity was enhanced in in vitro cultures of several mammalian cells by treatment with chitin and its derivatives. As a result, connective tissue formation was stimulated, and the self-defence function against microbial infection was enhanced at the cellular level. On the basis of these results, several chitin and chitosan dressing materials have been developed commercially for the healing treatment of human and animal wounds [59].

Chitosan is non-toxic and easily bioabsorbable with gel-forming ability at low pH. Moreover, chitosan has antacid and antiulcer activities which prevent or weaken drug irritation in the stomach. Also, chitosan matrix formulations appear to float and gradually swell in an acid medium. All these interesting properties of chitosan make this natural polymer an ideal candidate for controlled drug release formulations [60].

4. Decellularization

Autologous grafts are "gold standard" for implantation. However, the most disadvantage of autologous is quantity. The number of autograft does not meet needs of patients. Homograft is greater than autograft but they cannot satisfy needs of patient. Many patients must wait for a long time to take a homogenous organ. Xenograft is the greatest but they can evoke serious immune reaction. So, one method developed to process homograft and xenograft is decellularization. Every tissue/organ concludes cells and extracellular matrix. Cells are structure and functional units of tissue/organ but cells are major antigen of tissue/organ. Extracellular matrix is many protein, polysaccharide, protoglycan released by cell. ECM plays an important role in mechanical support, signal transportation, adherence of tissue/organ. Decellularization is a multi-step process to remove all cell components from tissue/organ and leave intact ECM. Many decellularization agents were researched such as physical methods, chemical methods and enzyme methods. Every decellularization agent has specific affections of cell and extracellular matrix. So, these agents are combined to make an effective decellularization process which removes all cell components and reverses maximum ECM. Decellularization effectiveness depends on type of tissue/organ. One agent can be a good detergent for decellularizing one tissue but not for another [61]. Moreover, cell derived ECM can be used as a matrix for cell culture.

Method	Mode of action	Effects on ECM
Physical		
Snap freezing	Intracellular ice crystals disrupt cell membrane	ECM can be disrupted or fracture during rapid freezing
Mechanical force	Pressure can burst cells and tissue removal eliminates cells	Mechanical force can cause damage to ECM
Mechanical agitation	Can cause cell lysis, but more commonly used to facilitate chemical exposure and cellular material removal	Aggressive agitation or sonication can disrupt ECM as the cellular material is removed
Chemical		
Alkaline; acid	Solubilize cytoplasmic components of cells; disrupts nucleic acids	Removes GAGs
Non-ionic detergents		
Triton X-100	Disrupts lipid–lipid and lipid–protein interactions, while leaving protein – protein interactions intact	Mixed results; efficiency dependent on tissue, removes GAGs
Ionic detergents		
Sodium dodecyl sulfate (SDS)	Solubilize cytoplasmic and nuclear cellular membranes; tend to denature proteins	Removes nuclear remnants and cytoplasmic proteins; tends to disrupt native tissue structure, remove GAGs and damage collagen
Sodium deoxycholate		More disruptive to tissue structure than SDS
Triton X-200		Yielded efficient cell removal when used with zwitterionic detergents
Zwitterionic detergents		
CHAPS	Exhibit properties of non-ionic and ionic detergents	Efficient cell removal with ECM disruption similar to that of Triton X-100
Sulfobetaine-10 and -16 (SB-10, SB-16)		Yielded cell removal and mild ECM disruption with Triton X-200
Tri(n-butyl)phosphate	Organic solvent that disrupts protein–protein interactions	Variable cell removal; loss of collagen content, although effect on mechanical properties was minimal
Hypotonic and hypertonic solutions	Cell lysis by osmotic shock	Efficient for cell lysis, but does not effectively remove the cellular remnants
EDTA, EGTA	Chelating agents that bind divalent metallic ions, thereby disrupting cell adhesion to ECM	No isolated exposure, typically used with enzymatic methods (e.g., trypsin)
Enzymatic		
Trypsin	Cleaves peptide bonds on the C-side of Arg and Lys	Prolonged exposure can disrupt ECM structure, removes laminin, fibronectin, elastin, and GAGs
Endonucleases	Catalyze the hydrolysis of the interior bonds of ribonucleotide and deoxyribonucleotide chains	Difficult to remove from the tissue and could invoke an immune response
Exonucleases	Catalyze the hydrolysis of the terminal bonds of ribonucleotide and deoxyribonucleotide chains	

Table 1. Overview of decellularization methods (Thomas W. Gilbert)

Today, many decellularization grafts were applied in clinical treatment such as acellular valve, vascular and some are commercial include: SurgisSIS (porcine small intestinal submicosa), Alloderm (human dermis), ACell (porcine urinary bladder)... Small intestine contains four layers such as mucosa, submucosa, muscularis externa and serosa. Small intestine submucosa (SIS) is a submucosa tissue between mucosa and muscularis externa. SIS is isolated from small intestine by mechanically removing of internal mucosal layer and outer muscular layer. Then, SIS is processed step-by-step with 0.1% peracid acid, 0.05% gentamycin and sterilized using 2500 kRad gamma irradiation. SIS is consisted of collagen, proteoglycan, glycosaminoglycan, glycoprotein and growth factor (VEGF, FGF-2 ...). Most of these components can be preserved in extracellular matrix after decellularizing. In tissue engineering, SIS is used as soft tissue grafts such as vascular, skin or used for reconstructing genitourinary, ligament tissue [62].

4.1. Vascular tissue engineering

Atherosclerosis is the most dangerous cardiovascular disease. Atherosclerosis is a condition in which vascular wall is harden, thicken because of fatty lipid accumulation. Atherosclerosis is responsible for millions of death all the world every year. In 2004, seventeen million people passed away because of cardiovascular disease all over the world (29% world total death). More than 7 million people are killed by coronary disease (9.6% world total death) (WHO). Heart American Association, in 2006, coronary disease was responsible for 17.6% death in America. One out of six American died for coronary disease [63].

Today, there are some methods to cure atherosclerosis including drug treatment, coronary artery bypass surgery and angioplasty. However, these methods can not cure this condition completely. More than 30% patients don't have qualified autogenous vascular grafts. Therefore, artificial grafts are made to overcome some current drawbacks.

Artifical graft can be classified into synthetic and biologic scaffold. Synthetic scaffolds include undegradable polymers such as Dacron, ePTFE and degradable polymers such as polylactic acid (PLA) and polyglycolic acid (PGA). Some advantages of synthetic polymers are easy processing, high initial strength, however, they have some disadvantages such as slow recellularization, poor ability to support remodeling. Biologic vascular grafts are either obtained by manipulating native proteins of vascular vessels such as collagen, elastin... or by decellularizing vascular vessels. Decellularized native vascular vessels have some advantages such as slow cost, reduction of graft rejection and immune reaction [64].

In the early time, decellularization studies were tested without cell-seeding. In 1990, Lantz et al use SIS (small intestine submucosa) as small-diameter arterial graft in18 dogs. 48 weeks after surgery, 28 vascular grafts (75%) were patent and tree dogs can survive from 76 to 82 weeks after implantation. This result suggested that small intestinal submucosa can be used in small diameter vascular tissue engineering [65]. In 2001, Hodde et al demonstrated that porcine SIS ECM extract containing vascular endothelial growth factor (VEGF) with concentration of 0.77 ng VEGF/g SIS [66]. In the same year, Nemcova et al isolated and decellularized SIS from bovine and porcine. Nine decellularized SIS grafts were implanted into femoral arteries of five male mongrel dogs. After 9 weeks, eight grafts remained patent and some kinds of cell such as endothelial cells (ECs), smooth muscle cells (SMCs) invaded into the grafts. No evidence of inflammatory and aneurysmal symptom was observed during the experimental time [67].

However, the main disadvantage of vascular graft is thrombus which ussually occurs immediately in vascular graft lumen after implantation. This process can lead to graft failure and threaten patients' survival. In order to solve this problem, ECs are used as anti-thrombus agent in vascular graft lumen, additionally, SMCs are used to improve mechanical strength of vascular graft. Broschel et al decellularized and recellularized rat iliac arterial grafts. Iliac arterial grafts were decellualrized by glycerin, SDS for 12 hours. Then, decellularized iliac grafts were recellularized with adult rat heart ECs and implanted to femoral arteries of allogeneic rats without systemic anticoagulation injection. After 4 weeks, 2 of 7 control grafts (29%) were patent (decellularized grafts without recellularization) and 8 of 9 (89%) experimental grafts (decellularized grafts with recellularization) maintained blood vessel patent [68]. Consequently, this experiment result proved excellent function of ECs in vascular tissue engineering. Some researchers on vascular tissue engineering seeded autologous vascular cells including ECs, SMCs and fibroblasts to make autologous tissue engineered vascular. At the same time, the appearance of bioreactor systems sped up development of vascular tissue engineering. Niklason developed a pulsatile perfusion bioreactor system in 2001. Bioreactor contained a stirbar, a lid for gas exchange and one (or two) silicone tubing(s). Porous vascular scaffolds were threaded over silicone tubing. Bovine aortic SMCs at the passage 2 or 3 were pipetted onto the outer surface of the scaffolds, then bioreactors were slowly rotated and removed to incubator with 10% CO_2, 100% humidity, and 37°C. Each silicone tubing was linked to a pulsatile perfusion system operated at 165 beats/minute and 260/-30 mmHg. After 8 weeks culture, under nonpulsatile condition, SMC growth was on the outer surface of tubing scaffold and poorly organized. Under pulsatile condition, SMC distribute homogenously in scaffold wall from outer to inner similar to native structure [69].

Nowaday, some decellularized vascular grafts can be obtained from human. Human umbilical veins and arteries can be used in decellularization experiment. Human umbilical arteries were isolated and completely decellularized by Gui et al in 2009. Decellularized umbilical arteries preserved intact collagen matrix and mechanical properties, burst pressure had no signicant change from native form. Decellularized artery graft remained patent after 8 weeks surgery [70]. In 2005, Joel Daniel et al processed human umbilical vein by automated dissection. Human umbilical cord was inserted a mandrel into vein and frozen to -20 and -80°C, human umbilical cord was maintained for 12 hours at least at this temperature. The mandrel was lathed with rotation speed of 2900 rpm, cutting depth of 750 μm. Then, human umbilical vein was decellularized with 1% (w/v) SDS. The result showed that the treated human umbilical vein contained no cell; burst pressure results were 972.8 ± 133.8 mmHg (972/1082), compliance results were 5.7 ± 1.3% over 80 – 120 mmHg. Vascular smooth muscle cells can adhere, proliferate and migrate on the surface of dHUV [71]. Tran Le Bao Ha et al carried out a research on decellularization method for HUVs. HUVs were isolated by manual dissection. HUVs were decellularized by distilled water or NaCl 3M or SDS 1%. The result confirmed that the combination between SDS 1% (24h) and NaCl 3M (24h) showed the best effective on cellular elimination.

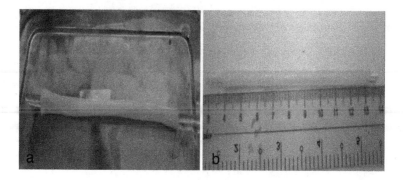

Figure 6. Human umbilical cord (a) and human umbilical vien (b)

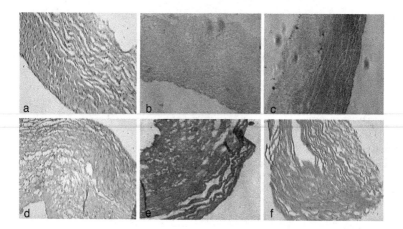

Figure 7. HE staining of HUV with different decellularization methods. Control (a), distilled water (b), NaCl 3M (c), SDS 1% 24h (d), SDS 1% 36h (e), SDS 1% 24. and NaCl 3M 24h (f)

4.2. ECM from cultured cells

One of the most important properties of ECM is its functional diversity. ECM has been reported to support and enhance for adhesion, migration, proliferation of cells as well as to create stem cell niches *in vitro.*. ECM can be harvested from different sources, one of which is from cells under culture condition. When cultured, cells will produce three-dimensional matrix surrounding themselves. A method is described for generating tissue culture surfaces coated with a human fibroblast-derived ECM [72, 73, 74, 75].

For this purpose, human foreskin fibroblasts are isolated, plated and cultured until third passage (see Figure 8). Fibroblasts are maintained in culture medium until reaching 80%

confluency and stimulated to synthesize ECM by culture medium supplemented ascorbic acid. Matrices are denuded of cells and cellular remnants are removed by using Triton X-100, NH$_4$OH and DNase.

Then, ECM coated culture surfaces are tested by staining with PI to access DNA remnant (see Figure 9), with H&E and PAS in order to characterize component of ECM. The results suggest that fibroblast-derived three-dimensional matrix was determined to be free of cellular constituents and still remain attached to the culture surface. The conducted matrices were washed and covered with PBS; and stored at 4⁰C. Under these conditions, biological activity (for example, induction of cell attachment, proliferation…) was reported to be well-preserved for up to 6 months.

In order to evaluate the quality of the ECM, the test of cell rapid attachment ability is performed. Cell proliferation on ECM is also assessed. Results showed that the cultured cells attached and proliferated on ECM coated surfaces faster than on ECM non-coated surfaces.

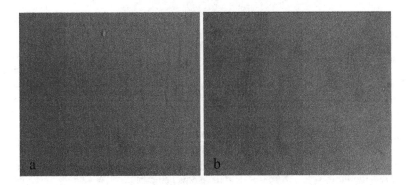

Figure 8. Fibroblasts are in cultured surfaces (a) and are stimulated to synthesize ECM (b)

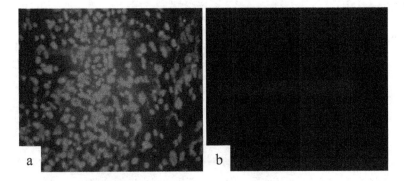

Figure 9. ECM stained PI before (a) and after (b) using DNase

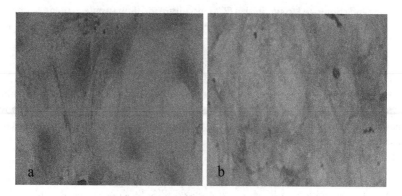

Figure 10. Culture surface before (a) and after (b) is denuded cells

5. Conclusion

In modern society, many diseases have been increasing in human because of pollution, accident, lifestyle... The mutilation in human body leads to expand the needs of replacing tissues/ organs. However, the available source of tissues/organs is limited. Creating artificial tissues/ organs for replacing damaged, dysfunctional tissues/organs becomes a big discipline on material science. Naturally derived biomaterials have been studied and applied in clinical applications as artificial tissues/organs because they are capable of supporting cell proliferation, biodegradability and remodeling tissues. Although the current results have not completely satisfy the clinical demand, the potential applications of naturally derived biomaterials are still highly considered, therefore, research on this field have now being taken place all over the world.

Author details

Tran Le Bao Ha[*], To Minh Quan, Doan Nguyen Vu and Do Minh Si

*Address all correspondence to: tlbha@hcmus.edu.vn

University of Science, Vietnam National University – Hochiminh city, Vietnam

References

[1] Lodish, H, Berk, A, & Zipursky, S. L. Molecular Cell Biology. New York: W. H. Freeman (2000).

[2] Anu, M. Type XV collagen. University of Oulu (2001).

[3] Hassan, N, Habibollah, P, & Abolhassan, A. Properties of the amniotic membrane for potential use in tissue engineering. European cells & materials (2008). , 15, 88-89.

[4] Andrew, H, Vijay, A. S, Trevor, G, Aaron, M. Y, James, L, David, K. J, & Harminder, S. D. Optimization of amniotic membrane (AM) denuding for tissue engineering. Tissue engineering (2008). , 14, 371-383.

[5] Singh, R, Purohit, S, & Chacharkar, M. P. Effect of high doses of gamma radiation on the functional characteristics of amniotic membrane. Radiation Physics and Chemistry (2007). , 76, 1026-1030.

[6] Loss, M, Wedler, V, Kunzi, W, Meuli-simmen, C, & Meyer, V. E. Artificial skin, split-thickness autograft and cultured autologous keratinocytes combined to treat a severe burn injury of 93% of TBSA. Burns (2000). , 26, 644-652.

[7] Ludwik, K. B, David, N. H, Mario, M. C, William, B. N, Oscar, E. M, & Marc, G. J. Amnion in the treatment of pediatric partial-thickness facial burns. Burns (2008). , 34, 393-399.

[8] Susan, S. Y. Current Protocols in Cell Biology. John Wiley & Sons, Inc. (2003). , 1-2.

[9] Rose, P. J, Mark, H. F, Bikales, N. M, Overberger, C. G, Menges, G, & Kroschwitz, J. I. editors. Encyclopedia of polymer science and engineering. New York, USA: Wiley (1989). , 488-513.

[10] Draget, K. I, Smidsrod, O, & Skjàk-bræk, G. Alginate from algae. In Polysaccharide and Polyamides in the food Industry. In: Steinbüchel A, Rhee SK. (eds). Wiley-VCH Verlag GmbH & Co.: Weinheim (2005). , 1-30.

[11] Ertesvåg, H, Valla, S, & Skjàk-bræk, G. Genetics and biosynthesis of alginates. Carbohyd. Europe (1996). , 14, 14-18.

[12] Paul, W, & Sharma, C. P. Chitosan and Alginate Wound Dressings: A Short Review. Trends in Biomaterials and Artificial Organs (2004). , 18, 18-23.

[13] Chen, J. P, Chu, I. M, Shiao, M. Y, Hsu, B. R, & Fu, S. H. Microencapsulation of islets in PEG amine modified alginate-poly(l-lysine)-alginate microcapsules for constructing bioartificial pancreas. Journal of Fermentation and Bioengineering (1998). , 86, 185-190.

[14] Rowley, J. A, Madlambayan, G, & Mooney, D. J. Alginate hydrogels as synthetic extracellular matrix materials. Biomaterials (1999). , 20, 45-53.

[15] Seifert, D. B, & Phillips, J. A. Porous alginate-poly(ethylene glycol) entrapment system for the cultivation of mammalian cells. Biotechnology progress (1997). , 13, 569-576.

[16] Altman, G. H. Silk-based biomaterials. Biomaterials (2003). , 24, 401-416.

[17] Tanaka, K, Inoue, S, & Mizuno, S. Hydrophobic interaction of containing Asn-linked oligosaccharide chains, with the H-L complex of silk fibroin produced by B. mori. Insect Biochemistry and Molecular Biology (1999)., 25.

[18] Inoue, S. Silk fibroin of Bombyx mori is secreted, assembling a high molecular mass elementary unit consisting of H-chain, L-chain, and with a 6:6:1 molar ratio. Journal of Biological Chemistry (2000)., 25.

[19] Seidel, A. Regenerated spider silk: Processing, properties, and structure. Macromolecules (2000)., 33, 775-780.

[20] Xu, M. Structure of a protein superfiber: spider dragline silk. Proceedings of the National Academy of Sciences of the United States of America (1990)., 87, 7120-7124.

[21] Kumaresan, P. Sericin a versatile by product. Indian Silk (2007)., 45, 11-13.

[22] Dandin, S. B. Biomedical uses of silk and its derivatives. Indian Silk (2007)., 45, 5-8.

[23] Gulrajani, M. L. Sericin-a bio-molecule of value. Indian Silk (2006)., 45, 16-22.

[24] Wang, Y. Cartilage tissue engineering with silk scaffolds and human articular chondrocytes. Biomaterials (2006)., 27, 4434-4442.

[25] Sofia, S. Functionalized silk-based biomaterials for bone formation. Journal of Biomedical Materials Research (2001)., 54, 139-148.

[26] Megeed, Z. Genetically engineered silk-elastinlike protein polymers for controlled drug delivery. Advanced drug delivery reviews (2002)., 54, 1075-1091.

[27] Medved, L. V, Gorkun, O. V, & Privalov, P. L. Structural organiza-tion of C-terminal parts of fibrinogen A alpha-chains. FEBS Lett (1983)., 160, 291-295.

[28] Ferry, J. D, & Morrison, P. R. Preparation and properties of serum and plasma proteins. VIII. The conversion of human fibrinogen to fibrin under various conditions. Journal of the American Chemical Society (1947)., 69, 388-400.

[29] Betts, L, Merenbloom, B. K, & Lord, S. T. The structure of fibrinogen fragment D with the 'A' knob peptide GPRVVE. Journal of Thrombosis and Haemostasis (2006)., 4, 1139-1141.

[30] Ryan, E. A, Mockros, L. F, Stern, A. M, & Lorand, L. Influence of a natural and a synthetic inhibitor of factor XIIIa on fibrin clot rheology. Biophysical Journal (1999)., 77, 2827-2836.

[31] Collet, J. P, Shuman, H, Ledger, R. E, Lee, S, & Weisel, J. W. The elasticity of an individual fibrin fiber in a clot. Proceedings of the National Academy of Sciences of the United States of America (2005)., 102, 9133-9137.

[32] Kaitlin, C, & Murphy, J. Kent Leach. A reproducible, high throughput method for fabricating fibrin gels. BMC Research Notes (2012).

[33] Bensaïd, W, Triffitt, J. T, Blanchat, C, Oudina, K, Sedel, L, & Petite, H. A biodegradable fibrin scaffold for mesenchymal stem cell transplantation. Biomaterials (2003). , 24, 2497-2502.

[34] Okada, M, & Blomback, B. Calcium and fibrin gel structure. Thrombosis Research (1983). , 29, 269-280.

[35] Siebenlist, K. R, & Mosesson, M. W. Progressive cross-linking of fibrin gamma chains increases resistance to fibrinolysis. Journal of Biological Chemistry (1994). , 269, 28414-28419.

[36] Alan, R. H, Dennis, K. G, Mark, P. H, Frank, C. S, & Constantine, E. Autologous Whole Plasma Fibrin Gel: Intraoperative Procurement. Archieves of Surgery (1992). , 127, 357-359.

[37] Ye, Q, Zünd, G, & Benedikt, P. Fibrin gel as a three dimensional matrix in cardiovascular tissue engineering. European Journal of Cardio-thoracic Surgery (2000). , 17, 587-591.

[38] Bensa, W, Triffittb, J. T, Blanchata, C, Oudinaa, K, Sedela, L, & Petitea, H. A biodegradable fibrin scaffold for mesenchymal stemcell transplantation. Biomaterials (2003). , 2497-2502.

[39] Saltz, R, Dimick, A, Harris, C, Grotting, J. C, Psillakis, J, & Vasconez, L. O. Application of autologous fibrin glue in burn wounds. Journal of Burn Care & Rehabilitation (1989). , 10, 504-507.

[40] Klemm, D, Philipp, B, Heinze, T, Heinze, U, & Wagenknecht, W. Comprehensive Cellulose Chemistry. Fundamentals and Analytical Methods. Wiley-VCH, Weinheim (1998).

[41] Myasoedova, V. V. Physical chemistry of non-aqueous solutions of cellulose and its derivatives. John Wiley and Sons, Chirchester (2000).

[42] Robert, J. M, Ashlie, M, John, N, John, S, & Je, Y. Cellulose nanomaterials review: structure, properties and nanocomposites. Chemical Society Reviews (2011). , 40, 3941-3994.

[43] Nabar, G. M, & Padmanabhan, C V. Studies in oxycellulose. Proceedings of the Indian Academy of Sciences (1950). , 31, 371-380.

[44] Kibbe, A. H. Handbook of pharmaceutical excipients: Cellulose, silicified microcrystalline. American Public Health Association. Washington (2000).

[45] Wadworth, L. C, & Daponte, D. Cellulose esters. In: Nevell TP, Zeronian SH (ed.) Cellulose Chemistry and its Applications. Ellis Horwood, Chich-ester (1985). , 349-362.

[46] Delgado, J. N, & William, A. Wilson and Gisvold's textbook of organic medicinal and pharmaceutical chemistry. Lippincott-Raven Publishers, Wickford (1998).

[47] Svensson, A, Nicklasson, E, Harrah, T, Panilaitis, B, Kaplan, D, Brittberg, M, & Gatenholm, P. Bacterial Cellulose as a Potential Scaffold for Tissue Engineering of Cartilage. Biomaterials (2005). , 26, 419-431.

[48] Muzzarellieditor. Natural Chelating Polymers. Pergamon Press, New York (1973).

[49] Zikakiseditor. Chitin, Chitosan and Related Enzymes. Academic Press, Orlando (1984).

[50] Dutta, P. K. Ravikumar MNV, Dutta J. Chitin and chitosan for versatile applications, Journal of Macromolecular Science-polymer Reviews (2002). , 42, 307-315.

[51] Kurita, K. Chemistry and application of chitin and chitosan, Polymer Degradation and Stability (1998). , 59, 117-120.

[52] Sashiwa, H, Shigemasa, Y, & Roy, R. Chemical modification of chitosan: synthesis of dendronized chitosan-sialic acid hybrid using convergent grafting of preassembled dendrons built on gallic acid and tri(ethylene glycol) backbone. Macromolocules (2001). , 34, 3905-3920.

[53] Baba, Y, Noma, H, Nakayama, R, & Matsushita, Y. Preparation of chitosan derivatives containing methylthiocarbamoyl and phenylthiocarbamoyl groups and their selective adsorption of copper (II) over iron (III). Analytical sciences (2002). , 18, 359-370.

[54] Qu, X, Wirsen, A, & Albertsson, A. C. Effect of lactic/glycolic acid side chains on the thermal degradation kinetics of chitosan derivatives. Polymer (2001). , 41, 4841-4850.

[55] Madhavan editor. Chitin Chitosan and their Novel Applications. Science Lecture Series, CIFT, Kochi (1992).

[56] Prasitslip, M, Jenwithisuk, R, Kongsuwan, K, Damrongchai, N, & Watts, P. Cellular responses to chitosan in vitro: the importance of deacetylation, Journal of Materials Science: Materials in Medicine (2000). , 11, 773-780.

[57] Lin, W. C, Liu, T. Y, & Yang, M. C. Hemocompatibility of polyacrylonitrile dialysis membrane immobilized with chitosan and heparin conjugate. Biomaterials (2003).

[58] Markey Bowman, Bergamini, editor. Chitin and Chitosan. Elsevier Applied Science, London (1989).

[59] Gebelein CarraherJr, editor. Industrial Biotechnological Polymers. Technomic, Lancaster (1995).

[60] Uhrich, K. E, Cannizzaro, S. M, Langer, R. L, & Shakesheff, K. M. Polymeric systems for controlled drug release. Chemical Reviews (1999). , 99, 3181-3190.

[61] Thomas, W. G. Decellularization of tissues and organs, Biomaterials (2006). , 27, 3675-3683.

[62] Jason, H. Naturally Occurring Scaffold for Soft Tissue Repair and Regeneration. Tissue Engineering (2002). , 8, 295-308.

[63] Véronique, L. R. Heart Disease and Stroke Statistics- (2012). Update: A Report from the Amercian Heart Association. Circulation 2012.

[64] Chrysanthi, W. Engineering of Small Diamter Vessels.Therapeutic applications: tissue therapy; , 1000-1013.

[65] Lantz Small Intestinal Submucosa as a Small-Diameter Arterial Graft in the Dog. Journal of Investigative Surgery (1990). , 3, 217-227.

[66] Hodde, J. P. Vascular endothelial growth factor in porcine-derived extracellular matrix. Endothelium (2001). , 8, 11-24.

[67] Nemcova, S, Noel, A. A, Jost, C. J, Gloviczki, P, Miller, V. M, & Brockbank, K. G. Evaluation of a xenogeneic acellular collagen matrix as a small-diameter vascular graft in dogs preliminary observations. Journal of Investigative Surgery (2001).

[68] Borschel, G. H. Tissue engineering of recellularized small-diameter vascular grafts. Tissue Engineering (2005). , 11, 778-786.

[69] Laura, E. N. Morphologic and mechanical characteristics of engineered bovine arteries. Journal of vascular surgery (2001). , 33, 628-638.

[70] Gui, L. Development of decellularized human umbilical arteries as small-diameter vascular grafts. Tissue Engineering (2009). , 15, 2665-2676.

[71] Joel, D. Development of the Human Umbilical Vein Scaffold for Cardiovascular Tissue Engineering Applications. ASAIO Journal (2005). , 51, 252-261.

[72] Kenneth, M. Y. Current Protocols in Cell Biology. John Wiley & Sons, Inc. (2003). , 1-10.

[73] Badylak, S, Gilbert, T, & Irvin, J. The extracellular matrix as a biologic scaffold for tissue engineering. Tissue Engineering (2008). , 121-144.

[74] Chen, R. N, Ho, H. O, Tsai, Y. T, & Sheu, M. T. Process development of an acellular dermal matrix (ADM) for biomedical application. Biomaterials (2004). , 25, 2679-2686.

[75] Cheng, Z. J, So, R. P, Byung, H. C, Kwideok, P, & Byoung, H. M. In vivo cartilage tissue engineering using a cell-derived extracellular matrix scaffold. Artificial Organs (2007). , 31, 183-192.

Chapter 4

Treatment of Bone Defects — Allogenic Platelet Gel and Autologous Bone Technique

Dragica Smrke, Primož Rožman, Matjaž Veselko and
Borut Gubina

Additional information is available at the end of the chapter

1. Introduction

Bone defects are a serious illness that can result after a pathological process has destroyed vital components of the bone. Most commonly the causative event is extensive trauma and subsequent infection. It can be also osteomyelitis that destroys the bone and leaves non-vital bone sequesters along the length of the bone. This damage to the bone and soft tissues heals slowly and restitution can be only expected after some time of rest and procedures of debridement.

1.1. Bone defects

Bone defect by definition is a lack of bone tissue in a body area, where bone should normally be. Lack of bone tissue results in a pseudarthrosis, artificial joint that has no physiological importance. In that area, two parts of diseased bone are joined with a fibrous tissue. That area also lacks appropriate vascularization and is usually covered with scarred or fibrotic skin [1].

Bone defects can be treated by various surgical methods. One is always constrained with fibrosis that healed a wound or the site of infection [2]. Often there are factors that impair bone healing like diabetes mellitus [3, 4], immunosuppressive therapy [5, 6], poor locomotory status and others that one has to take in account when a procedure is planned.

There are some common methods of bone defect reconstruction, like decortication, excision and fixation, cancellous bone grafting [7] and the Ilizarov intercalary bone transport method [1]. The application of these methods results in successful final outcomes as far as the bone restitution is concerned.

However, one must consider repeated surgical procedures and often long hospitalization time or frequent outpatient visits for these patients. It is also common for patients to have prolonged ambulatory impairment with suboptimal functional and aesthetic results [8, 9].

1.2. Tissue bioengineering

Tissue engineering involves the restoration of tissue structure or function through the use of living cells. The general process consists of cell isolation and proliferation, followed by a re-implantation procedure in which a scaffold material is used. Cell sources can be autologous or allogenic cells. Autologous cells are usually the better choice, because the allogenic cells could incite immune rejection by the recipient. Mesenchymal stem cells provide a good alternative to cells from mature tissue and have a number of advantages as a cell source for bone and cartilage tissue regeneration [10].

Some authors report that most tissue engineering applications in the head and neck area would probably involve the use of chondrocytes and osteoblasts along with some type of scaffold material because of the importance of initial support and shaping [11].

Theoretically, the ideal bone graft substitutes should be osteogenic, biocompatible, bioabsorbable, able to provide structural support, easy to use clinically and cost-effective. A composite graft combines an osteoconductive matrix with bioactive agents that provide osteoinductive and osteogenic properties [12].

Novel techniques have been studied recently, many involving growth enhancers with varying results. These have been used for healing wounds, ulcers, fractures, and in maxillofacial settings. Such biological enhancers are autologous platelet rich plasma (PRP) in the form of activated platelet gel and recombinant bone morphogenetic proteins (rBMP) [11, 13-23]. An animal study showed enhanced bone growth when autologous bone was combined with platelet-rich plasma [24, 25].

The healing effects of platelet rich gel were attributed to the numerous growth factors (GFs) released by the platelets after activation [19, 26]. Some of those identified are: the platelet derived growth factor (PDGF), TGF-α and β (transforming growth factor alpha and beta), EGF (epidermal growth factor), FGF (fibroblast growth factor), IGF (insulin growth factor), PDEGF (platelet derived epidermal growth factor), PDAF (platelet derived angiogenesis factor), IL-8 (interleukin-8), TNF-α (tumour necrosis factor alpha), CTGR (connective tissue growth factor), GM-CSF (granulocyte macrophage colony stimulating factor), KGF (keratinocyte growth factor), and Ang-2 (angiopoetin), as reviewed by several authors [26, 27]. The inductive potential of platelet gel in tissue regeneration could also be attributed to its significant antimicrobial activity [28].

1.3. Clinical experiments

Recent studies on patients for the regeneration of long bone and foot and ankle defects have provided promising clinical results when using platelets as a source of GFs [10]. Some studies demonstrated that with the use of platelet gel a better and stronger bone yield was achieved as compared to reconstruction with conventional methods [29]. X-ray images of treated bones showed increased density early in follow up and in-growth of treated area was enhanced [30].

In the majority of clinical experiments, authors have applied autologous platelets obtained by preoperative apheresis from the peripheral blood of the patient undergoing surgery. However, this may not always be the best solution. In cases of diabetes it has been shown that the release of platelet GFs is decreased in experimental diabetic animals [31]. If allogeneic platelet rich plasma was used as a source of additional GFs, healing of tissues in diabetic patients can considerably improve [32].

Allogenic single donor platelet units are easy to obtain, since they are a standard blood bank product. They are highly standardized in terms of platelet content and residual leukocyte and red blood cell content is low. All of this is due to proven centrifugal forces used for their isolation, temperature of centrifugation, techniques of separation and processing and composition of preservative solution. Also, they are available in large quantities and considered safe. Autologous platelet preparations, on the other hand, are subject to enormous variability, which hinders serious studies of their clinical efficacy [33].

We used for our procedures the standard blood bank platelet concentrates. We prepared a graft composed of allogeneic platelet gel mixed with autologous cancellous bone in order to improve the healing conditions in bone defects, which was successfully demonstrated in our pilot clinical case [34].

In our case study, we showed that the healing potential of the gel GFs obtained from a high number of allogeneic platelets could be combined with the bone forming potential of autologous osteogenic and other stem cells from the cancellous bone. We employed the plasticity of the resulting graft mixture for the modeling and all of this contributed to a successful clinical outcome.

2. Body

2.1. Problem statement

The treatment of bone defects of long bones after injury is still one of the most difficult tasks in reconstructive bone surgery. The golden standard in bone graft surgery is still the use of autologous bone graft [7]. In certain settings, especially in extensive bone defects, this method of treatment could be insufficient and could only pose an additional trauma for the patient.

Numerous authors have reported difficulties when treating defected non-unions, such as extremely long healing time and incorporation of the graft, necrosis of the grafts, and reacutisation of infection [35, 36]. Concomitantly, long-term immobilization contributed to the contractures of the joints and soft tissue, and in the long-term perspective, also to the inferior functional and aesthetic results [37].

Pseudarthroses with certain mid size bone defect are complicated to treat because it is difficult to determine an appropriate treatment method. Smaller size defects can be treated with simple bone fixation and some debridement. Larger bone defects must be treated with bone transport (Ilizarov method) or transplant of bone graft with vascular pedicle [36].

Reconstruction by vascularised bone transfer along the Ilizarov intercalary bone transport and cancellous bone grafting has been the most widely used method of treatment for large defected nonunions after injury [37, 38]. There have been several modifications of the Ilizarov method, which retain its versatility, stability and mechanics, but these methods also contribute to a high rate of complications [35, 37, 38].

Mid sized defects can be treated with cancellous bone transplant, but many limitations exist with this method. Cancellous bone is of limited availability in human body and sometimes sources have been depleted after repeated surgeries. Often, resorption of transplanted cancellous bone is seen which leads to unsuccessful bone defect bridging [39].

Bone grafts are used to replace a part of the bony defect or to enhance the healing of a fracture. Because of the inability to procure large quantities of autologous bone and the added morbidity for the patient associated with the autograft donor site, new methods of bone transplant materials have emerged in recent years [7].

Substitutes for bone defects have been tested and one of the research tasks is to devise a easily attainable promotor of ingrowth of autologous cancellous bone. Theoretically, the ideal bone graft substitutes should be osteogenic, biocompatible, bioabsorbable, able to provide structural support, easy to use clinically and cost-effective. A composite graft combines an osteoconductive matrix with bioactive agents that provide osteoinductive and osteogenic properties [39].

Synthetic substitutes that provide a scaffold to support or direct bone formation include calcium sulphate, ceramics, calcium phosphate, cements, collagen, bioactive glass and synthetic polymers. These are available in a variety of formulations, including pellets, cement and injectable paste [39, 40].

The functional properties of bone morphogenetic proteins (BMP) 2 and 7, mesenchymal stem cells (MSC), demineralised bone matrix, and biocompatibile ceramics are presented in many papers describing their use in bone defect treatment [41-44]. Bone morphogenetic proteins exhibit an extraordinary power to induce new bone formation de novo without the presence of cancellous bone [45]. With their high cost, limited availability and restricted clinical indications, BMPs are a less attractive option for clinical application.

One of the clinical challenges in long bone defects is the induction of appropriate bone formation, especially in patients with diabetes. Several studies have demonstrated the clinical efficacy of various platelet derived GFs. Recent evidence shows that in diabetic patients platelets are handicapped by decreased expression of growth factors and lower potential for healing fractures [31, 46].

Although there is some evidence that the GFs are released to some extent in the stored platelet concentrates, the majority of GFs remain intact in the platelet granules if they are appropriately stored for up to 5 days [47].

The safety and efficacy of allogeneic platelets was also shown in our recent pilot case study [34]. Moreover, the preparation of autologous platelet gel requires pre-operative apheresis and blood draws from the patient, and adds to the complexity, risk and cost of surgery [48].

Based on these facts, we were of the opinion that allogeneic platelets constitute a superior alternative to autologous preparations obtained by pre-operative apheresis. Therefore, we used a standard platelet concentrate from the blood bank as a component for the activated platelet gel.

2.2. Application area

Tissue engineering involves the restoration of tissue structure or function through the use of living cells. The general process consists of cell isolation and proliferation, followed by a re-implantation procedure in which a scaffold material is used. Cell sources can be autologous or allogenic cells.

Autologous cells are usually the better choice, because the allogenic cells could incite immune rejection by the recipient. Mesenchymal stem cells are progenitor cells and can be developed in a laboratory along separate cell families. They can be differentiated into more maturated cells like osteoblasts and chondroblasts and chondrocytes. They provide a good alternative to cells from mature tissue and have a number of advantages as a cell source for bone and cartilage tissue regeneration [49].

Here we present the results of a prospective clinical study performed from May 2004 to February 2010 in the University Clinical Centre Ljubljana, Slovenia. We treated defected non-union of long bones with cancellous bone transplantation. We used allogeneic platelets as a source of additional GFs.

We treated 9 consecutive patients (3 female and 6 male), aged from 21 to 73 years (average 45.9 years), each with a defect of a different long bone (3 femoral, 4 tibial, 1 humeral and 1 ulnar). We present patients' size of bone defect, which were classified as mid-size in a Table 1.

Patient	Pseudarthrosis site	Graft volume in mL
1	Femur	16
2	Distal tibia	35
3	Distal tibia	45
4	Femur	15
5	Distal tibia	30
6	Proximal femur	25
7	Humerus	35
8	Ulna	30
9	Distal tibia	25
	Average graft volume	28.5

Table 1. Size of bone defect per patient and average of the group

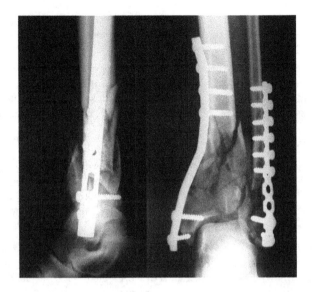

Figure 1. Bone defect of distal tibia (plain X-ray)

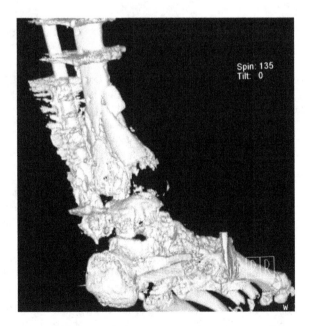

Figure 2. Bone defect of distal tibia CT reconstruction

They had already been unsuccessfully treated with conventional methods in our or other hospitals. The therapeutic options in these cases had been exhausted. In the Figure 1 and 2, we present an example of a bone defect we treated.

In 2 of the patients, we treated osteomyelitis before applying our treatment. We took additional microbiological samples at the time of operation. Three samples were positive for pathologic bacteria and patients received appropriate antibiotic therapy. After the operation no reacutisation of infection was noted. Two of the patients had diabetes on per oral therapy.

2.3. Research course

In our clinical investigation plan, the primary objective was to establish the potency of allogeneic platelet gel, from our blood bank, added to the transplanted autologous cancellous bone when treating post-traumatic mid-sized bone defect, with a follow-up of one year. The secondary objective was to investigate the healing, safety, handling and tolerance of the method and potential cost benefits.

We noted all the patients' major variables in a protocol, radiologic examinations, and postoperative follow-up for up to one year. As a survey of the immunological side effects of allogeneic platelets, we performed a screening of HLA antibodies class I and human platelet antibodies (HPA) before the implant operation and in the third month after the operation.

2.4. Methods used

We harvested autologous cancellous bone from one or both patients' iliac crests and ground it by hand and instruments until the particles were smaller than 5 mm. It was then stored on a sterile dish with wet gauze for later use.

For preparation of the platelet gel we used a standard allogeneic random single donor platelet concentrate that was ABO and RhD matched, serologically HIV, HBV, HCV and lues-negative, leukocyte depleted, and irradiated. A standard single donor platelet concentrate was prepared from 450 mL of whole blood, containing 70×10^9 platelets in 50 mL of citrated plasma, and stored in a plastic bag designed for platelet storage at 20-24ºC on an automatic agitator for up to five days.

We performed leukocyte depletion by using a commercial filter (BioP05 Plus, Fresenius HemoCare, Bad Homburg, Germany) with 10–15% platelet loss post-filtration. We irradiated the platelet concentrate with a cobalt irradiator with 25 Gray. All platelet related procedures, including the bacteriological controls, were performed according to the recommendations for blood banking procedures.

Finally, we prepared a mixture of lightly compressed autologous cancellous bone and an equal volume of allogeneic platelet concentrate with approximately 1.4×10^9 platelets per 1 mL (which is around five times higher than the physiological level of platelets in the blood).

We mixed the ingredients and added the fibrin glue components (human thrombin (100 IU/mL) in 40mM $CaCl_2$ (Beriplast P, ZLB Behring, Marburg, Germany)) for the activation of platelets and polymerization of fibrinogen. The implant is presented in the Figure 3. The mixture achieved the appropriate plasticity in 20 to 30 seconds. The resulting gelatinous graft was shaped according to the defect and implanted.

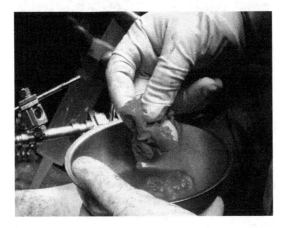

Figure 3. Cancellous bone and platelet rich plasma implant

2.5. Surgical procedure

In all our operations, we approached the bone defects through previous surgical incisions after administering a single dose of prophylactic antibiotic. After debridement of the non-union which is presented in Figure 4, we filled the resulting bone defect with a semi-solid, moldable gelatinous graft, presented in the Figure 5.

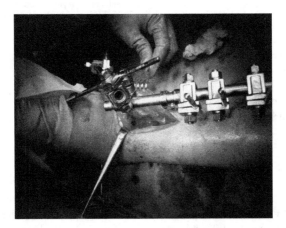

Figure 4. Bone defect at the operation

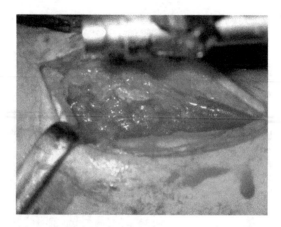

Figure 5. Bone defect filled with implant

We revised the method of fracture fixation and repositioned bone fragments were and fixed them in good alignment. We applied a different fixation method where it was necessary or inadequate and we present the fixation methods in Table 2.

Patient	Pseudarthrosis site	Fixation method
1	Femur	Internal plate
2	Distal tibia	External fixator
3	Distal tibia	Internal plate
4	Femur	Tutor brace
5	Distal tibia	Internal plate
6	Proximal femur	Dynamic hip screw with long plate
7	Humerus	Internal plate
8	Ulna	External fixator
9	Distal tibia	Internal plate

Table 2. Fixation methods used and graft volume per patient

We placed negative pressure suction subcutaneously, away from the graft in order to minimize the removal of GFs. All procedures were carried out within a sterile operation field - aseptic conditions.

In the follow-up protocol, we assessed the general status after the operation, and the bone configuration with X-ray at 2, 4, 6, and 12 months. We assessed bone remodeling at 6 and 12 months by CT scan. We drew blood samples from each patient at week 14 for the identification of anti-HLA/Class I antibodies and anti-HPA antibodies in order to assess potential immune reactions related to the use of allogeneic platelets. We used the standard in-house platelet immuno-fluorescence test (PIFT) and antigen capture ELISA test (PAK-12, GTI, Brookfield, USA) to screen for antibodies.

2.6. Results

We removed the drains on the second or third day after the operation, draining different volumes, on average 250 mL (200 to 450 mL). Immediate post-operative care was uneventful in all cases. We discharged the patients 6-8 days after the operation and they were regularly examined in the outpatients' clinic.

Out of 9 patients, 7 successfully healed their defect with the implant (78%). Figure 6 shows healed bone defect in distal tibia.

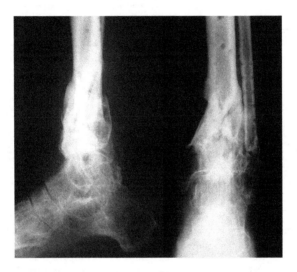

Figure 6. Healed bone defect after grafting and platelet additive

Different healing times are presented in Table 3.

Time in weeks	Minimal	Maximal	Average	Median
Time to appearance of hazy callus	6	24	10	8
Time of partial weight bearing	12	40	22.5	18
Time of free mobility and full weight bearing	16	48	31	31
Time of overall bone healing	16	36	23	24

Table 3. Healing times after the operation for successful cases (time in weeks)

We noted major complications during the treatment in 3 patients (33%): poor incorporation of implant, mental deterioration leading to non-compliance, and radial nerve palsy, which receded (1 patient respectively). Two of these patients had to undergo further surgery. More detailed data of bone healing are displayed in Table 4.

Patient /sex/age (years)	Time to appearance of hazy callus (weeks)	Time to partial weight bearing in defects (weeks)	Time to free mobility and full weight bearing (weeks)	Extent of graft incorporation	Time to stable bone healing (weeks)	Complications during treatment	Major compli- cation	Final result (12 months)
1/F/63	8	12	40	complete	16	none	no	healed
2/M/50	8	18	32	proximally 1/4, distally complete	24	left hip fracture	no	healed
3/F/49	10	16	-	complete proximally, distally not at all	24	pseudarthrosis, re-operated	yes	failed
4/M/45	24	32	44	both ends 1/2	28	none	no	healed
5/F/45	8	40	48	proximally ½, distally not at all	36	poor compliance, mental disorder, pseudarthrosis, re-operated	yes	failed
6/M/73	6	16	24	complete	24	extremity shortening	no	healed
7/M/33	8	-	16	complete	16	n. radialis paresis	yes	healed
8/M/21	12	-	16	complete	16	none	no	healed
9/M/34	8	18	30	complete	24	none	no	healed

Table 4. Detailed bone healing data

No side effects caused by the implant were observed; no platelet or HLA-class I antibodies were detected in any patient on follow-up.

We observed the survival of the implant to be excellent; most of the volume of the implant was preserved. Of clinical importance are ingrowths of the implant into adjacent bone. This was critical in the case of distal tibia (patient 2, 3, 5, and 9), where we observed diminished incorporation in the distal part, where the metaphysis of the tibia is less vascularized. In the case of femur pseudarthrosis (patient 6), bone quality was insufficient for the implant to regenerate the whole bone circumference, so healing was prolonged.

In theory, allogeneic platelets could have several certain side effects. In order to minimize these, all platelet units in our study were leuko-depleted and irradiated in order to prevent immune and bacteriological side effects, especially alloimmunisation to HLA-Class I and HPA antigens [50]. In fact, there was no evidence of immune reactions or transfusion-transmitted infections following the procedures. There have been no signs of bacterial contamination, which is not strange, based on the recent observation that the platelet gel exhibits significant antimicrobial activity in vitro [28].

The combined autologous/allogeneic graft showed successful incorporation into the defective pseudarthrosis in 7 out of 9 patients, which was confirmed with the CT scans and plain X-ray film. The problem with the two patients in whom the therapy failed was the poor incorporation of the graft in the distal tibia, where bone healing is compromised through many factors [51].

One of the patients had a deteriorating psychiatric disorder and could not follow instructions later in the study, and one had a poor bone situation arising from previous treatments. The other seven patients with successful outcomes achieved a satisfactory clinical improvement with no side effects related to the procedure.

A bacterial infection did not reoccur in cases where an infection was previously treated. Our treatment has concluded prolonged ongoing hospitalizations and immobilizations for some patients who previously underwent numerous operations and rehabilitations. Only one patient had to be reoperated only once again, because of poor implant ingrowth.

2.7. Further research

As bioengineering techniques improve and become more clinically applicable, so does the field of application expand. In our work we have shown one of the methods to be useful in treating mid-size bone defects.

Further application of platelet rich plasma as a source of growth factors can be used in other settings where tissue defects exist. It is a natural derivative like blood transfusion and can be applied on the part of the body, where natural mechanisms would need some bioengineering support.

Further investigation should be directed into measuring the comparative efficiency of this treatment. It should be compared to golden standard treatment and determine also novel applications in bigger and smaller defects.

3. Conclusion

We showed that adding a platelet gel to a cancellous bone graft can help in retaining grafted bone from resorption and enhances its incorporation into adjacent bone. The standard platelet concentrates from the blood bank did not pose a significant risk for the affected patient. The results indicate good reasons for the application of this method in the treatment of bone defects in long bones.

This is the first report of a prospective clinical study monitoring the use of allogeneic platelets mixed with autologous cancellous bone for the treatment of the non-union of long bones after fractures. Our new method of tissue engineering seems to have the potential to become a widely approved and accepted method of bone tissue replacement in the treatment of the non-union of long bones.

Last, but not least, it is worth noticing that the outdate rate of the platelet units is currently in the range of 8-27% of all prepared platelet units [52] This leads to the conclusion that the successful use of allogeneic platelets would significantly decrease the amount of wasted platelets, which could consequently favorably change the results of blood banking policies.

Acknowledgements

This work was partly supported by research grants J3-6290 and P3-0371 from the Slovenian Research Agency, ARRS, Trg OF 13, SI-1000 Ljubljana, Slovenia. No private company or pharmaceutical company funded this project.

Author details

Dragica Smrke[1], Primož Rožman[2], Matjaž Veselko[1] and Borut Gubina[1*]

*Address all correspondence to: gubina@gmail.com

1 Department of Surgery, University Medical Center Ljubljana, Ljubljana, Slovenia

2 Blood Transfusion Centre of Slovenia, Ljubljana, Slovenia

References

[1] Gordon, L, & Chiu, E. J. Treatment of infected non-unions and segmental defects of the tibia with staged microvascular muscle transplantation and bone-grafting. J Bone Joint Surg Am, (1988). , 377-386.

[2] Longo, U. G, et al. Tissue engineered strategies for pseudoarthrosis. Open Orthop J, (2012). , 564-570.

[3] Follak, N, Kloting, I, & Merk, H. Influence of diabetic metabolic state on fracture healing in spontaneously diabetic rats. Diabetes Metab Res Rev, (2005). , 288-296.

[4] Lu, H, et al. Diabetes interferes with the bone formation by affecting the expression of transcription factors that regulate osteoblast differentiation. Endocrinology, (2003). , 346-352.

[5] Boddenberg, U. Healing time of foot and ankle fractures in patients with diabetes mellitus: literature review and report on own cases]. Zentralbl Chir, (2004). , 453-459.

[6] Kagel, E. M, & Einhorn, T. A. Alterations of fracture healing in the diabetic condition. Iowa Orthop J, (1996). , 147-152.

[7] Sen, M. K, & Miclau, T. Autologous iliac crest bone graft: should it still be the gold standard for treating nonunions? Injury, (2007). Suppl 1: , S75-S80.

[8] Cattaneo, R, Catagni, M, & Johnson, E. E. The treatment of infected nonunions and segmental defects of the tibia by the methods of Ilizarov. Clin Orthop Relat Res, (1992). , 143-152.

[9] Smrke, D, & Arnez, Z. M. Treatment of extensive bone and soft tissue defects of the lower limb by traction and free-flap transfer. Injury, (2000). , 153-162.

[10] Kitoh, H, et al. Transplantation of marrow-derived mesenchymal stem cells and platelet-rich plasma during distraction osteogenesis--a preliminary result of three cases. Bone, (2004). , 892-898.

[11] Henderson, J. L, et al. The effects of autologous platelet gel on wound healing. Ear Nose Throat J, (2003). , 598-602.

[12] Malhotra, A, et al. Can platelet-rich plasma (PRP) improve bone healing? A comparison between the theory and experimental outcomes. Arch Orthop Trauma Surg, (2013). , 153-165.

[13] Fisher, D. M, et al. Preclinical and Clinical Studies on the use of Growth Factors for Bone Repair: A Systematic Review. Curr Stem Cell Res Ther, (2013).

[14] Bhanot, S, & Alex, J. C. Current applications of platelet gels in facial plastic surgery. Facial Plast Surg, (2002). , 27-33.

[15] Carlson, N. E, & Roach, R. B. Jr., Platelet-rich plasma: clinical applications in dentistry. J Am Dent Assoc, (2002). , 1383-1386.

[16] Crovetti, G, et al. Platelet gel for healing cutaneous chronic wounds. Transfus Apher Sci, (2004). , 145-151.

[17] Dugrillon, A, et al. Autologous concentrated platelet-rich plasma (cPRP) for local application in bone regeneration. Int J Oral Maxillofac Surg, (2002). , 615-619.

[18] Englert, S. J, Estep, T. H, & Ellis-stoll, C. C. Autologous platelet gel applications during cardiovascular surgery: effect on wound healing. J Extra Corpor Technol, (2005). , 148-152.

[19] Franchini, M, et al. Efficacy of platelet gel in reconstructive bone surgery. Orthopedics, (2005). , 161-163.

[20] Fuerst, G, et al. Enhanced bone-to-implant contact by platelet-released growth factors in mandibular cortical bone: a histomorphometric study in minipigs. Int J Oral Maxillofac Implants, (2003). , 685-690.

[21] Gandhi, A, et al. The role of platelet-rich plasma in foot and ankle surgery. Foot Ankle Clin, (2005). viii., 621-637.

[22] Giannoudis, P. V, & Einhorn, T. A. Bone morphogenetic proteins in musculoskeletal medicine. Injury, (2009). Suppl 3: , S1-S3.

[23] Kain, M. S, & Einhorn, T. A. Recombinant human bone morphogenetic proteins in the treatment of fractures. Foot Ankle Clin, (2005). viii., 639-650.

[24] Li, G. Y, et al. Efficacy of leukocyte- and platelet-rich plasma gel (L-PRP gel) in treating osteomyelitis in a rabbit model. J Orthop Res, (2012).

[25] Hakimi, M, et al. Combined use of platelet-rich plasma and autologous bone grafts in the treatment of long bone defects in mini-pigs. Injury, (2010).

[26] Frechette, J. P, Martineau, I, & Gagnon, G. Platelet-rich plasmas: growth factor content and roles in wound healing. J Dent Res, (2005). , 434-439.

[27] Westerhuis, R. J, Van Bezooijen, R. L, & Kloen, P. Use of bone morphogenetic proteins in traumatology. Injury, (2005). , 1405-1412.

[28] Bielecki, T. M, et al. Antibacterial effect of autologous platelet gel enriched with growth factors and other active substances: an in vitro study. J Bone Joint Surg Br, (2007). , 417-420.

[29] Yamada, Y, et al. Tissue-engineered injectable bone regeneration for osseointegrated dental implants. Clin Oral Implants Res, (2004). , 589-597.

[30] Fontana, S, et al. Effect of platelet-rich plasma on the peri-implant bone response: an experimental study. Implant Dent, (2004). , 73-78.

[31] Tyndall, W. A, et al. Decreased platelet derived growth factor expression during fracture healing in diabetic animals. Clin Orthop Relat Res, (2003). , 319-330.

[32] Gandhi, A, et al. The effects of local insulin delivery on diabetic fracture healing. Bone, (2005). , 482-490.

[33] Borzini, P, & Mazzucco, L. Tissue regeneration and in loco administration of platelet derivatives: clinical outcome, heterogeneous products, and heterogeneity of the effector mechanisms. Transfusion, (2005). , 1759-1767.

[34] Smrke, D, et al. Allogeneic platelet gel with autologous cancellous bone graft for the treatment of a large bone defect. Eur Surg Res, (2007). , 170-174.

[35] Smrke, D, & Arnez, Z. M. Case of severe injury of lower limb treated with new Ljubljana traction method. Injury, (1999). , 501-503.

[36] Karlstrom, G, & Olerud, S. Fractures of the tibial shaft; a critical evaluation of treatment alternatives. Clin Orthop Relat Res, (1974). , 82-115.

[37] Paley, D, et al. Ilizarov treatment of tibial nonunions with bone loss. Clin Orthop Relat Res, (1989). , 146-165.

[38] Green, S. A, et al. Management of segmental defects by the Ilizarov intercalary bone transport method. Clin Orthop Relat Res, (1992). , 136-142.

[39] Bollo, A, & Lewis, J. Different forms of bone grafts. J Foot Ankle Surg, (1996). , 400-405.

[40] Lind, M, & Bunger, C. Factors stimulating bone formation. Eur Spine J, (2001). Suppl 2: , S102-S109.

[41] Calori, G. M, et al. Bone morphogenetic proteins and tissue engineering: future directions. Injury, (2009). Supplement 3): , S67-S76.

[42] Giannoudis, P. V. Fracture healing and bone regeneration: autologous bone grafting
or BMPs? Injury, (2009). , 1243-1244.

[43] Griffin, X. L, Smith, C. M, & Costa, M. L. The clinical use of platelet-rich plasma in
the promotion of bone healing: a systematic review. Injury, (2009). , 158-162.

[44] Ranly, D. M, et al. Platelet-rich plasma inhibits demineralized bone matrix-induced
bone formation in nude mice. J Bone Joint Surg Am, (2007). , 139-147.

[45] Forriol, F, et al. Platelet-rich plasma, rhOP-1 (rhBMP-7) and frozen rib allograft for
the reconstruction of bony mandibular defects in sheep. A pilot experimental study.
Injury, (2009). Suppl 3: , S44-S49.

[46] Gandhi, A, et al. The effects of local platelet rich plasma delivery on diabetic fracture
healing. Bone, (2006). , 540-546.

[47] Valeri, C. R, Saleem, B, & Ragno, G. Release of platelet-derived growth factors and
proliferation of fibroblasts in the releasates from platelets stored in the liquid state at
22 degrees C after stimulation with agonists. Transfusion, (2006). , 225-229.

[48] Calori, G. M, et al. Application of rhBMP-7 and platelet-rich plasma in the treatment
of long bone non-unions: a prospective randomised clinical study on 120 patients. Injury, (2008). , 1391-1402.

[49] Pittenger, M. F, et al. Multilineage potential of adult human mesenchymal stem cells.
Science, (1999). , 143-147.

[50] Brand, A. Immunological aspects of blood transfusions. Transpl Immunol, (2002). ,
183-190.

[51] Ristiniemi, J. External fixation of tibial pilon fractures and fracture healing. Acta Orthop Suppl, (2007). , 3.

[52] Nightingale, S, et al. Use of sentinel sites for daily monitoring of the US blood supply. Transfusion, (2003). , 364-372.

Chapter 5

Skeletal Muscle Ventricles (SMVs) and Biomechanical Hearts (BMHs) with a Self-Endothelializing Titanized Blood Contacting Surface

Norbert W. Guldner, Peter Klapproth,
Hangörg Zimmermann and Hans- H. Sievers

Additional information is available at the end of the chapter

1. Introduction

For most patients with end-stage heart failure (more than 90%) there is no definitive treatment option up to now. This fact is caused on the one hand by a severe shortage in donor hearts, and on the other hand by technical and economic limitations of mechanical cardiac assist devices and artificial hearts. An additional cardiac output of 2-3 litres per minute should give most patients with end-stage heart failure a better quality of life and a longer survival. Latissimus dorsi muscle as a source for muscular blood pumps would have several advantages. Its availability is nearly unlimited, there is no foreign tissue rejection and of course no need for an immune-suppression, less risk of infection and this procedure should be less costly than heart transplantation and the treatment with fully implantable cardiac assist devices and artificial hearts.

Skeletal muscle ventricles (SMVs) and Biomechanical Hearts (BMHs) are experimental muscular blood pumps to support the circulation. They are developed and tested as future treatment option for patients with end stage heart failure. SMVs and BMHs basically have two main limitations: firstly muscle damage after electrical muscle fiber transformation from a fast twitched into a slow twitched non-fatigue muscle and secondly thromboembolic complications from the blood contacting surface especially when a muscular blood pump works on demand. Former investigators developed sack-ventricles within circulation in dogs pumping up to 4 years [1-5].

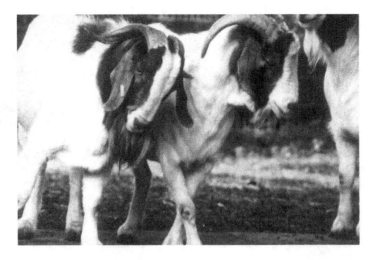

Figure 1. Boer goats with a weight between 60 and 100 kg and a latissimus dorsi muscle of 300 to 450 g.

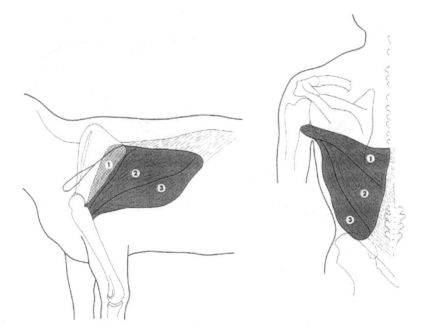

Figure 2. Topography of the latissimus dorsi muscle (LDM) in a big animal (goat) and a human. LDM consists of three parts: Pars transversalis (1), Pars obliqua (2) and Pars lateralis (3), LDMs weight is 300 to 450g in Boer bocks and about 600g in humans.

2. Training device

To study muscle protection of LDM under different stimulation patterns and drugs to improve muscular power an elastic training device was created, where the LDM was wrapped around and muscle performance could become evaluated [6].

The training device (Figure 3) is made of silicone rubber (Q3, Dow Corning). It consists of a central chamber and two compliant side bladders filled with saline solution. The barrel-shaped central chamber and the side bladders have volumes of 150 mL and 50 mL each, respectively. The side bladders are constructed with a compliance of 1.0 to 1.3 mL/mmHg, simulating the windkessel characteristics of the arterial system in normal subjects with 1.07 mL/mmHg. More technical details can be found elsewhere (Guldner et al.,1994; 2000).

Elastic Training Device

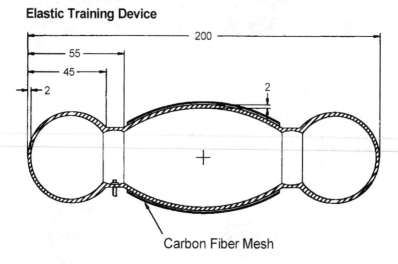

Carbon Fiber Mesh

Figure 3. The Frog, an elastic training device, made of silicone, consists of a central pumping chamber which is compressible but not extendible (carbon fibre mesh).

3. Intra-thoracic implantation

Experiments were carried out in adult Boer goats (Figure 1), with a weight of 70±11 kg. They were castrated 4 weeks before the operation to keep them together and avoid injuries between them. The experiments were performed in accordance with the Guide for the Care and Use of Laboratory Animals published by the National Institutes of Health. They were supervised by a representative of the District President of the local society for Prevention of Cruelty to Animals.

The operation was performed under general anaesthesia. Left LDM was dissected free, folded to a double layer, and wrapped around the central chamber of the training device. The SMV was transferred into the thorax and fixed at the thoracic wall.

Commercially available myostimulators were used (Medtronic model 7420/7424 and Telectronics model 7220). An epi-mysial electrode 30mm long (custom-made, Medtronics, Bakken Research Center) was attached to the muscle close to the branches of the nervus thoracodorsalis. On the opposite side of the muscle, an electrode 60mm long (Medtronics SP 5591 – 500-60-NMS) was placed sub-fascially.

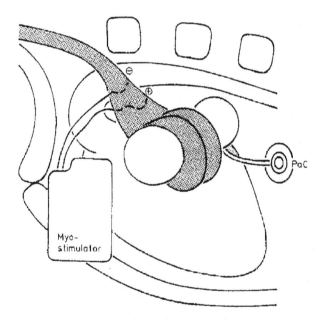

Figure 4. An intra-thoracic skeletal muscle ventricle is wrapped around the Frog: A myostimulator induces muscle contractions via 2 electrodes. Contractions of LDM cause a volume shift from the central chamber into the expanding bladders, with a corresponding pressure increase. This pressure is measured by piercing a subcutaneous vascular access port (PaC).

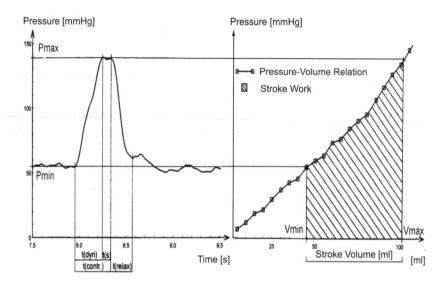

Figure 5. Method of stroke volume and stroke energy determination, relating pressure increase of a ventricle contraction (left) to the compliance curve of the bladders of the Frog, stroke volume is received (right). The area of the stroke volume below the compliance curve represents the stroke work or stroke energy [7].

Stroke volume evaluation is performed relating maximal pressure P_{max} from the pressure curve during muscle contraction to the compliance curve of the Frog's elastic side bladders (Figure 5). Stroke volume multiplied with P_{max} results in stroke work W. Daily energy in KJ/d is to calculate by stroke work W multiplied with the number of SMV contractions per day.

4. Clenbuterol supported dynamic training of skeletal muscle ventricles against systemic load

The profound loss of power that occurs in skeletal muscle after electrical conditioning has been the major limiting factor in its clinical application. This study investigates a 3-fold approach for chronic conditioning of skeletal muscle ventricles combining electrical transformation, dynamic training against systemic load and pharmacological support with clenbuterol.

In 10 adult male goats, SMVs were constructed from latissimus dorsi wrapped around an intrathoracic training device with windkessel characteristics [8]. SMVs were stimulated electrically and trained dynamically by shifting volume against systemic load. Group 1 goats were controls (n=5), and group 2 goats (n=5) were supported with clenbuterol (150µg 3 times a week).

Peak pressure, stroke volume and stroke work per day were significantly improved (p< 0.007) in the clebuterol- treated group after 151±2.7 days (Fig. 6). At termination, myosin heavy chains were totally transformed into myosin heavy chain-I in all SMVs. Other investigators found different functional and histological effects of clenbuterol in dogs [9].

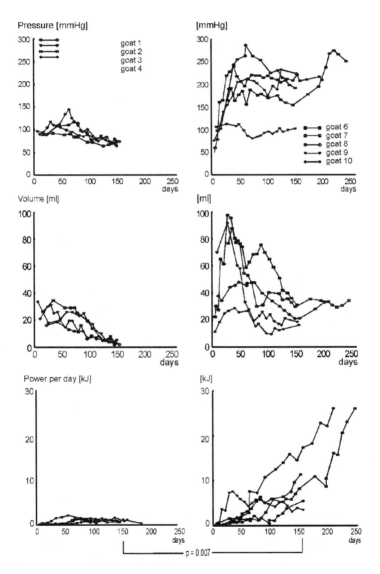

Figure 6. Time course of systolic pressure (top), stroke volume (middle), and power per day (bottom) during dynamic training of SMVs without Clenbuterol n=5 (left) and supported by clenbuterol n=5 (right) against load conditions of 60 to 70 mm Hg [8].

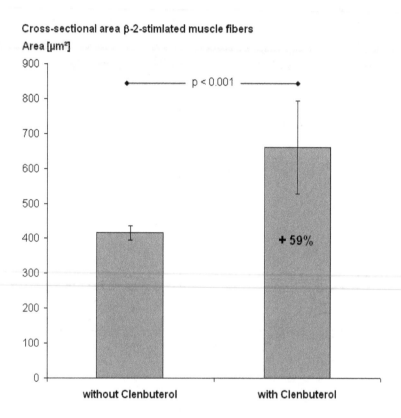

Cross-sectional area β-2-stimlated muscle fibers

Figure 7. Cross-section areas of clenbuterol treated (β-2-stimulated) muscle fibers were enhanced by 59%.

5. Fibertransformation preserving non-fatiguable Typ IIa fibers

In our experience muscular blood pumps that were active over several months, were highly vulnerable when totally transformed into type I muscle showing severe muscle damage and decreased function. Thus, in our new experimental setting, encouraged by the Liverpool findings of the working group of Salmons and Jarvis [10], fast and fatigue resistant muscle ventricles were performed around the Frog. Pre-stimulation with about 2 Hz proceeded in situ, to open intramuscular collaterals connecting the proximal with the distal blood supply of the muscle and to increase capillary density. Thereafter we used continuous basic burst stimulation with an average pulses frequency of less than 1 Hz. Intermittent series of pumping within the Frog were performed, measuring pumping capacity in correlation to stimulation frequency. This procedure should be a "model setting" for a pumping on demand. During our first investigations, we could see that intermittent pumping capacity was already manifold after 4 to 5 months of pumping (Figure 8).

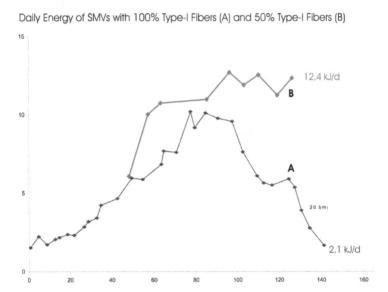

Daily Energy of SMVs with 100% Type-I Fibers (A) and 50% Type-I Fibers (B)

Figure 8. Daily energy of goat A (lower curve) with a mean pulse frequency of 5 Hz, which is massively declined. With 1 Hz stimulation in goat B however (upper curve) a high pumping capacity was observed.

Mean electrical pulse frequency with 5 Hz of group A (n=6) in Fig.9 resulted in a non relevant delivery of daily energy after 200 days of pumping. A 1 Hz stimulation of group B however showed an enhancing pressure and stroke volume and an increasing development of daily energy after 200 days with a well preserved muscular tissue.

Gel electrophoresis for myosin heavy chains MHC I and MHC IIa analysis (Figure 10) of group A with a mean pulse frequency of 5Hz showed a composition of MHC I (bottom of the gel) and MHC IIa (top of the gel) with mainly MHC IIa in the controls (C). In the trained SMVs (T) of group A was 100% MHC-I in all cases. In group B and with 1 Hz stimulation over months MHCIIa was preserved (50% MHC-IIa and 50% MHC-I). The preservation of Type II MHC in group B explains the more powerful contractions and the maintained pressure, stroke volume and daily energy (Figure 9).

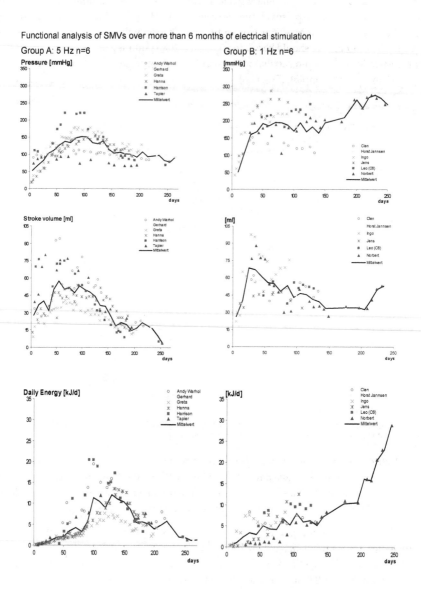

Figure 9. Systolic pressure (top), stroke volume (middle) and daily energy (bottom) of group A (n=6) with a mean pulse frequency of 5 Hz (left) and with 1 Hz in group B (n=6, right).

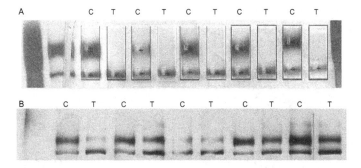

Figure 10. Gel electrophoresis of myosin heavy chains MHC I and MHC IIa from group A with a mean pulse frequency of 5 Hz. Control (C) was the non stimulated contra-lateral LDM. In group B with a mean stimulation frequency of 1 Hz, type IIa MHC is well preserved and about 50% after several months in all stimulated SMVs.

6. Stroke volume of SMVs with 100% type-I-fiber (A) vs. SMVs with 50% type-IIa fiber (B)

As an example one fast, relatively fatigue resistant SMV delivered a maximal pump volume of about 3 L/min. It could be maintained over two minutes. Thereafter it decreased to 1,5 L/min after 5 minutes. This dynamic adaptation of stroke volume per minute in that high level of pumping volume up to 3 L/min was solely possible in the 50% type IIa fibre muscle. 100 % type I fibre ventricles did enhance its pumping capacity however only up to 1 L/min.

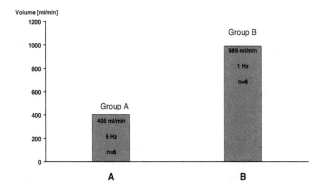

Figure 11. Stroke volumes evaluated in a Frog surrounded by a goat's SMV of a latissimus dorsi muscle of 330g up to 200 days postoperatively. In group A with 100% type I fibres stroke volume per minute was at 405 ml and in the fast, relatively fatigue resistant muscle with about 50% type IIa fibres stroke volume per minute was at 888 ml per minute. This amount of stroke volume per minute could be maintained over months.

Stroke Volume on Demand [ml/min]

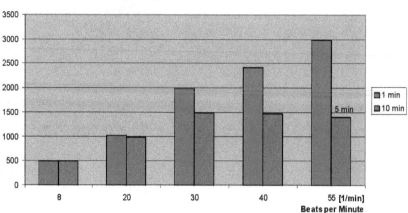

Figure 12. Stroke volumes of an "on demand" setting (see text!) evaluated in a Frog surrounded by a goat's SMV of a latissimus dorsi muscle of 330g 6 weeks postoperatively.

These recent experimental results in SMVs around the Frog were basic to construct a preclinical Biomechanical Heart Model on demand, which is described as follows.

7. Valve-less Biomechanical Hearts

Biomechanical Hearts, constructed in adult Boer goats (n=5), are blood pumps, consisting of a pumping chamber with clinically relevant stroke volumes [11]. They can be integrated into the circulation in a one-step operative procedure during pharmacological stimulation with the β-2-stimulator Clenbuterol (5 x150µg/wk). This experimental pumping chamber, made of PTFE, was anastomosed to the descending aorta by two ring armoured PTFE-prostheses (Impra Medica GmbH, München), as shown in Figure 13. The pumping chamber was used mainly for three reasons: firstly, to stabilize the ventricular pump cavity with improved flow characteristics to minimize thrombo-embolic complications; secondly, to prevent muscle damage by overstretch-induced ischemia; and thirdly, to prevent a ventricular chamber rupture.

During surgery, the mean stroke volume of BMHs was 53.8±22.4 ml. One month after surgery, in peripheral pressure, the mean and minimal diastolic pressure of BMH-supported heart cycle differed significantly from unsupported ones (Figure 14). After BMH-supported heart contractions, the subsequent maximal rate of pressure generation, dP/dt $_{max}$ increased by 20.5±8.1% (p<0.02). One BMH, catheterized 132 days after surgery, shifted a volume of 34.8 mL per beat and 1.4 L/min with a latissimus dorsi muscle of 330 g (Figure 14, top).

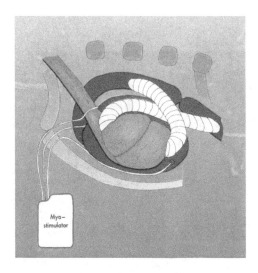

Figure 13. Scheme of an experimental setting in a big animal model in an aorto-aortic configuration. The thoracic aorta is ligated between the two anastomoses. Two muscular stimulation electrodes activate the LDM and an epicardial sensing electrode enables the syncronization with the heart cycle.

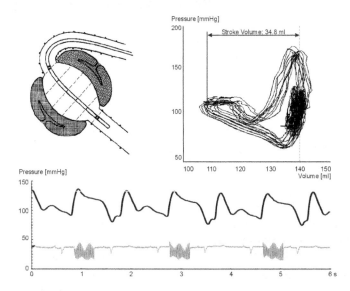

Figure 14. Stroke volume determination with a conductance catheter, placed within the pumping chamber of the BMH (left, top). Pressure-volume-loop of a BMH on postoperative day 132 with a stroke volume of 34.8 ml and an output of 1400ml per minute (right, top). ECG with stimulation bursts, a pressure trace from a peripheral artery where the BMH is in a 1:2 mode and synchronized with the heart (bottom).

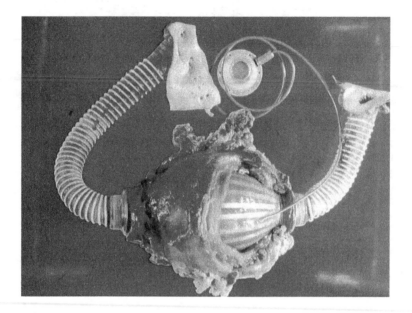

Figure 15. Explanted BMH without valves after 414 days of pumping within a Boer goat. The pumping chamber was made of a double layered polyurethane membrane including steel springs and it was connected to the aorta by ring armoured PTFE prostheses.

8. Hemodynamic evaluations of a valve equipped Biomechanic Heart Model supporting a failing myocardium in goats

As shown previously in goats, valve-less Biomechanical Hearts (BMHs) of a clinically relevant size could be trained effectively in the systemic circulation under support of clenbuterol. Pumping capacity was more than 1 L/min but due to a high pendulum volume no significant flow contribution for the circulation was gained. Thus, the following investigations were performed to evaluate the efficacy of valve-equipped BMHs in comparison to valve-less BMHs. To mimic the clinical situation, this test was performed in failing hearts [12].

Heart failure was induced in adult Boer goats (n=5) by a repeated intra-coronary embolization. A valve-bearing and balloon-equipped pumping chamber was integrated into the descending aorta simulating standardized circulatory BMH support. Circulatory flow was evaluated by a flow meter around the pulmonary artery. Myocardial function was evaluated by a conductance catheter placed in the left heart ventricle (Figure 16).

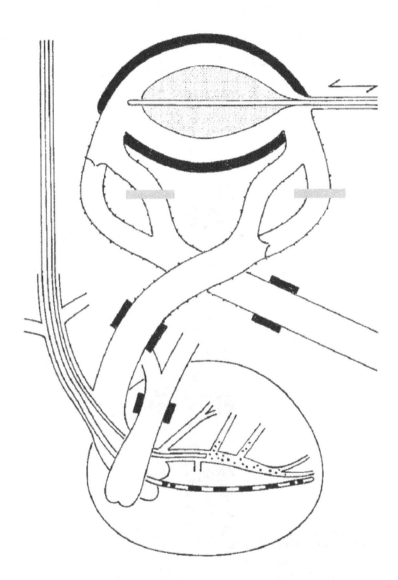

Figure 16. BMH model is made of a stiff polyurethane chamber with an integrated pumping balloon. The dividing and re-uniting vascular prostheses were connected end –to-end with the divided descending aorta. In this setting two of the four prosthetic limbs carried heart valves. Thus, by clamping, no, one or two valves could be integrated into the circulation. The influence of different valve configurations on circulation could be evaluated in supporting a failing heart. Ultrasonic flow probes were placed around the pulmonary artery, aortic arch and the descending aorta. Within the left heart ventricle a conductance catheter was placed, and via a catheter within the left coronary artery an embolization could be induced and a flow wire could be introduced [12].

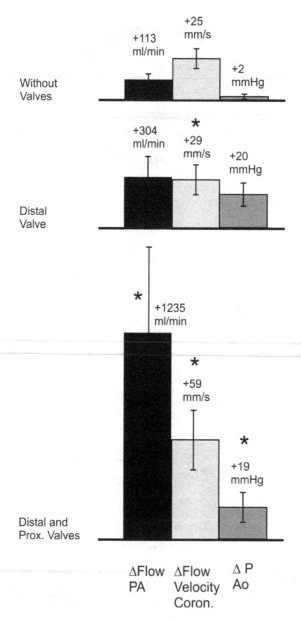

Figure 17. Results of the BMH model described in Fig. 16, without, with a distal and with two valves: mean aortic pressure(P_{Ao}, grey column), mean pulmonary flow (Q_{PA}, black column), mean flow velocity within the left coronary artery (V_C, white column) [12].

Valve-less BMHs offered an additional pulmonary flow of 113± 37 ml/min resp. 5.4±1.8%, those with one distal valve offered 304±126 ml/min resp. 14.5±6%. BMHs equipped with two valves increased the pulmonary blood flow by 1235± 526 ml/min resp. 58±25 % (p<0.05), the mean aortic pressure in this setting raised to 19±9 mmHg (p<0.05) and the coronary flow velocity to 59±18 mm/sec (p<0.05). Corresponding reduction of left ventricle's end-diastolic pressure ranged from 31 to 17 mmHg (p<0.05), while the myocardial dp/dt increased by 470±192 mmHg/s resp. 145±48 % (p<0.05).

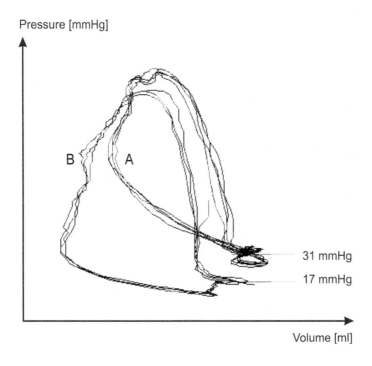

Figure 18. PV- loops from a conductance catheter placed in the left heart ventriclea cavum, without (A) and with an activated (B) double-valved BMH-model as shown in Figure16. It works ECG-triggered in a 1:2 mode with a balloon inflation of 60ml helium gas. The area within a loop represents the left heart ventricles stroke work. During activation of the BMH-model the stroke work of the failing heart ventricle is increased (B) and the end-diastolic pressure (LVEDP) drops from 28 to 14 mmHg [12].

The use of two valves in BMHs is essential for a relevant circulatory support. Unloading and contractility of the left heart ventricle were thus improved significantly. Two-valves-BMHs driven by a sufficient skeletal muscle ventricle may contribute to the therapy of a failing myocardium.

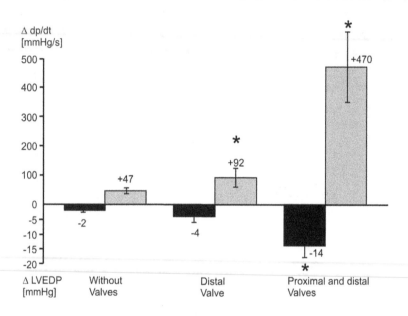

Figure 19. Reduction of the left ventricular end-diastolic pressure (LVEDP, black columns) evaluated as demonstrated in Figure 16 and 18 and an increase of the left ventricular contractility activation of the pumping balloon from the BMH-model in Figure 16, without, with a distal and with a proximal and a distal valve.

9. Valve equipped Biomechanical Hearts

As demonstrated above, efficacy of BMHs on the circulation is dependent on the integration of two heart valve prostheses into the in- and outflow part of the pumping chamber. Valve equipped Biomechanical Hearts were constructed and integrated within circulation in adult Boer goat (n=5), and pharmacological stimulation with the β-2-stimulator Clenbuterol. (5X150μg/wk). This pumping chamber, made of PTFE, was anastomosed to the descending aorta by two ring armoured PTFE-prostheses (Impra Medica GmbH, München). Between these prostheses two porcine glutaraldehyde fixed valve bearing porcine aortic conduits were integrated like shown in Figure 20.

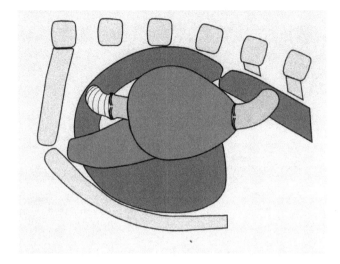

Figure 20. Scheme of an experimental setting from a valve equipped Biomechanical Heart in a big animal model (Boer goats) in an aorto-aortic configuration. The thoracic aorta is ligated between the two anastomoses. Two porcine glutaraldehyde fixed valve bearing porcine aortic conduits were integrated between the connecting PTFE prostheses and the PTFE pump ventricle.

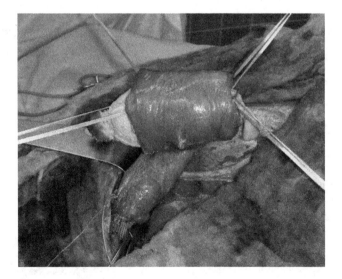

Figure 21. Operative situs of a BMH before transferring it into the cavity of the thorax, with four strings to fix it via the thoracic wall to the inner thoracic surface. Two stimulation electrodes and an artificial muscle tendon made of Dacron for a re-fixation onto the external thoracic wall are visible.

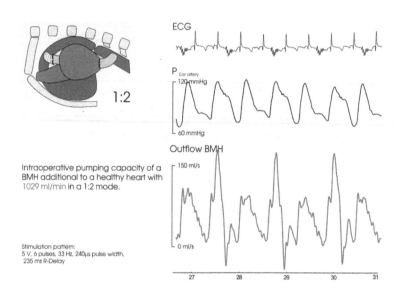

Figure 22. Intraoperative testing of the function of a valve equipped BMH by visualization of burst stimulation within the ECG, a 1:2 support within the arterial pressure curve and the flow curve which was obtained by a flow probe around the distal biologic aortic conduit

	Stroke Volume (L/ min)	Type of pumping chamber	Days of Pumping	Days of Survival	MHC-I	Significant Findings and Cause of Death
Larry	1029,6	Dacron	93	93	56 %	Seroma in both pleura
Juan	407,5	Dacron	267	301	95 %	Acute abdomen, total thrombosis of the pumping chamber, sacrification
Ugo	444,5	Dacron	136	182	78 %	Acute abdomen, total thrombosis of the pumping chamber, sacrification
Stanley	474,9	ePTFE (titanized)	225	385	94 %	Hematothorax, bleeding from proximal conduit, no chamber thrombus formation
Pierre	588	ePTFE (titanized)	180	446	100 %	Acute abdomen, intestinal infection, no chamber thrombus formation
Valeri	576,3	ePTFE (titanized)	531	914	--	Infection, sepsis. no chamber thrombus formation

Table 1. Intra- and post-operative data of six experimental valve equipped BMHs in adult Boer Goats

10. Self-endothelializing titanized blood contacting surface for Biomechanical Hearts

Titanium has proven itself as the leading structured metallic biomaterial for 50 years [13]. One reason for this widespread use is the excellent biocompatibility of the metal and its alloys [14]. Theoretically, surface coating of the blood contacting PTFE may open new avenues for improving biocompatibility of this kind of implant material. However, a titanium coating on PTFE seemed not to be possible until now due to the high temperatures needed for commonly used sputtering techniques. Therefore a novel coating method was used [15] for PTFE applying a plasma activated chemical gas deposition (PACVD) at temperatures of 30-35°C.

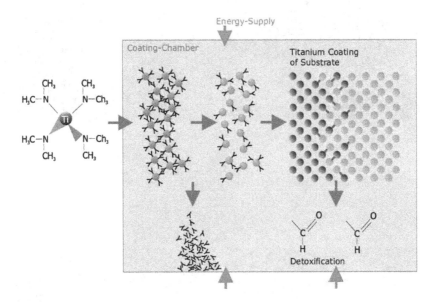

Figure 23. Principle of titanium coating at low temperature (see text).

PACVD is a coating technology (Pfm Titanium GmbH, Nürnberg, Germany, patent number EP 0 897 997 A1) where the so called precursor (Tetrakisdimethylamidotitanium, Ti $[N(CH_3)_2]_4$) is transferred into the gas phase and brought into the reactor by a carrier gas like nitrogen gas [16]. The plasma is able to supply the substrate with high energy while the temperature during deposition can be kept low at about 30-35°C. Within that non-thermal plasma with high electron temperatures but neutrons and ions at room temperature, solely the electrons can follow a quickly changing electrical field with a typical frequency of 13.56 MHz under low pressure plasma as described in detail elsewhere [17]. The precursor, or part of it, reacts with the substrate and creates a layer of 30nm in thickness (Figure 23).

The blood contacting surface of the PTFE-made pumping chamber was titanized as described above. This titan surface attracts progenitor cells derived from the bone marrow which were delivered into circulation. The seeded cells transform into endothelial cells within time [18]. This kind of self-tissue engineering of the blood contacting surface is mandatory to prevent thrombo-embolism mainly for blood pumps contracting on demand [14].

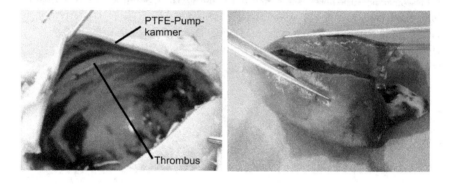

Figure 24. Thrombosis of the total blood contacting surface 8 weeks after implantation (left): Isolated thrombus formation from the PTFE- pumping chamber (right).

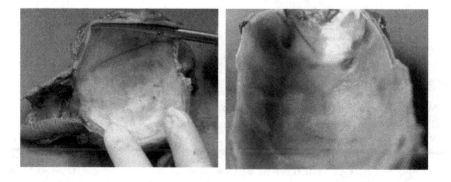

Figure 25. Titanized PTFE pumping chamber 6.5 months after implantation without any thrombus formation. This thin cover could be identified as an endothelial layer by a von Willebrand immun-histological staining.

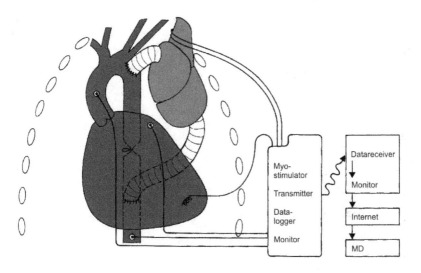

Figure 26. Clinical setting of a BMH in an aorto-aortic configuration

11. Summary and perspectives

A BMH is therapeutically indicated for patients with end-stage heart failure with an additional need of a support with 2-3 litres per minute "on demand", especially for candidates older than 60 years having no chance for heart transplantation. For a severe bi-ventricular myocardial insufficiency however, heart transplantation is the first choice.

Experimental Biomechanical Hearts in Boer goats with autologous skeletal muscle were to construct pumping up to 1.400 mL/min for more than 400 days under support of Clenbuterol. Furthermore was to demonstrate that a BMH model supporting a failing heart in Boer goats could pump about 2 litre blood per minute additionally. BMHs equipped with two valves were most effective in-vivo. Effective circulatory support by counter pulsation was achieved by SMVs elsewhere [19].

Muscle damage and power-loss of a BMH can be avoided by a muscle protective myostimulator applying a closed-loop controlled stimulation and thus maintaining type IIa fibres over years (Microstim GmbH, MyoSen®, Wismar; Germany). A titanized blood contacting surface with endothelialization (Pfm titanium GmbH, Nürnberg; Germany) might prevent thromboembolic complications. In the light of 25 years of systematic progress in basic science of muscle powered cardiac assist this biologic treatment option should become reconsidered as a future surgical treatment option for the therapy of end-stage heart failure [20].

Acknowledgements

We thank Prof. Dr. Petra Margaritoff, Hamburg University of Applied Sciences, Germany for critical reading of the manuscript.

Author details

Norbert W. Guldner[1], Peter Klapproth[2], Hangörg Zimmermann[3] and Hans- H. Sievers[1]

*Address all correspondence to: Guldner@uni-luebeck.de

1 Clinic of Cardiac Surgery, University of Lübeck, Germany

2 Microstim GmbH, Wismar, Germany

3 Pfm Titan GmbH Nürnberg, Hangörg Zimmermann, Germany

References

[1] Acker MA, Hammond RL, Mannion JD, Salmons S, Stephenson LW. Skeletal muscle as the potential power source for a cardiovascular pump: assessment in vivo Science 236 (1987), 324-327.

[2] Bridges Jr. CR, Brown WE, Hammond RL, Anderson DR, Anderson WA, DiMeo F, Stephenson LW. Skeletal muscle ventricles: Improved performance at physiologic preloads . Surgery 106 (1989), 275-28.

[3] Hooper TL, Niinami H, Hammond RL, Lu H, Ruggiero R, Pochettino A, Stephenson LW. Skeletal muscle ventricles as left atrial-aortic pumps: short-term studies . Ann Thorac Surg 1992;54:316-322.

[4] Lu H, Fietsam R, Jr., Hammond RL, Nakajima H, Mocek FW, Thomas GA, Ruggiero R, Colson M, Stephenson LW. Skeletal muscle ventricles: left ventricular apex to aorta configuration . Ann Thorac Surg 1993;55:78-85.

[5] Thomas GA, Hammond RL, Greer K. Functional assessment of skeletal muscle ventricles after pumping for up to four years in circulation. Ann Thorac Surg 2000; 70 (4): 1281-1289.

[6] Guldner NW, Eichstaedt HC, Klapproth P, Tilmans MHJ, Thuaudet S, Umbrain V, Ruck K, Wyffels E, Bruyland M, Sigmund M, Messmer BJ, Bardos P. Dynamic training of skeletal muscle ventricles. A method to increase muscular power for cardiac assistance. Circulation 89 (3):1032-1040 (1994).

[7] Klapproth P, Guldner NW, Sievers HH. Stroke volume validation and energy evalu-
     ation for the dynamic training of skeletal muscle ventricles. Int.J Artif Organs 1997;
     20:313-21.

[8] Guldner NW, Klapproth P, Großherr M, Rumpel E, Noel R, Sievers HH. Clenbuterol
     supported Dynamic Training of Skeletal Muscle Ventricles Against Systemic Load- A
     Key for Powerful Circulatory Assist ? Circulation 101:2213-2219 (2000)

[9] Sharif Z, Hammond RL, Mc Donald P, Vander Heide R, Stephenson LW. The func-
     tional and histological effects of clenbuterol on the canine skeletal muscle ventricle. J
     Surg Res. 123, 89-95 (2005)

[10] Lopez-Guajardo A, Sutherland H, Jarvis JC, Salmons S. Induction of a fatigue-resist-
     ant phenotype in rabbit fast muscle by small daily amounts of stimulation. J Appl
     Physiol. 2001; 90 (5):1909-18

[11] Guldner NW, Klapproth P, Großherr M., Rumpel E, Noel R, Sievers HH. Biomechan-
     ical Hearts: Muscular Blood Pumps, Performed in a One-Step Operation, and
     Trained under Support of Clenbuterol, Circulation 2001;104 717-22.

[12] Guldner NW, Klapproth P, Margaritoff PRJ, Noel R, Sievers HH, Großherr M. The
     Impact of Valves in a Biomechanical Heart Model Assisting Failing Hearts. Asian
     Cardiovasc Thorac Ann 2009;17:1-6

[13] Sivaram S. Chemical vapor deposition: thermal and plasma deposition of electronic
     materials.Van Nostrand Reinhold, New York. 1995.

[14] Dag B. (Ed.) Surface Characterization.Wiley-VCH, Weinheim. 1997.

[15] Guldner NW, Jasmund I, Zimmermann H, Heinlein M, Girndt B, Meier V, Flüß F,
     Rohde D, Gebert A, Sievers HH. Detoxification and Endothelialization of Glutaralde-
     hyde-Fixed   Bovine   Pericardium   With   Titanium   Coating;   Circulation;
     2009;119:1653-1660

[16] Brunette DM. Titanium in medicine. Springer, Berlin, Germany. 2001.

[17] Sedelnikov N, Cikirikicioglu M, Osorio-Da Cruz S, Khabiri E, Donmez Antal A, Tille
     JC, Karaca S, Hess OM, Kalangos A, Walpoth B. Titanium coating improves neo-en-
     dothelialisation of ePTFE grafts. Thorac Cardiovasc Surg. 2006; 54 suppl 1: 83-115.

[18] Guldner NW, Jasmund I, Zimmermann H, Heinlein M, Girndt B, Großherr M, Klin-
     ger A,Sievers HH. The First Self-Endothelialized Titanium Coated Glutaraldehyde-
     Fixed Heart Valve Prosthesis within Systemic Circulation.J Thorac Cardiovasc Surg
     2009, 138: 248-25

[19] Ramnarine IR, Capoccia M, Ashley Z, Sutherland H, Salmons S, Jarvis JC. Counter-
     pulsation From the Skeletal Muscle Ventricle and the Intraaortic Ballon Pump in the
     Normal and Failing Circulations. Circulation. 114 [suppl I]: 1-15 (2006)

[20] Salmons S. Cardiac assistance from skeletal muscle: a reappraisal. Europ J of Cardio
     thoracic Surg 35, 204-213 (2009)

Chapter 6

Fabrication of PGA/PLA Scaffold with the Shape of Human Nose

Qiong Li, Lu Zhang, Guangdong Zhou, Wei Liu and
Yilin Cao

Additional information is available at the end of the chapter

1. Introduction

Reconstructive surgery for the repair of nose deformities is challenging [1]. Nasal surgery involves autologous rib or septum cartilage grafts [2] and prosthetic devices [3] for reconstruction and reinforcement of the nasal skeleton. These conventional procedures are associated with donor site morbidity, limited tissue availability, and prosthesis related infection and extrusion [4]. Although tissue engineering is a promising method for repair and reconstruction of cartilage defects [5- 7], engineering cartilage with a delicate three dimensional (3D) structure, such as human nose, remains a great challenge in this field. Since in 1997 Cao *et al.* engineered the cartilage with a shape of human auricle in a nude mouse model [8], many researchers have tried to explore further developments of this tissue engineering system, but few of them have succeeded in *in vitro* regeneration of a cartilage construct with a complete and anatomically refined structure [9].

One major reason leading to the failure of *in vitro* engineering a cartilage construct with sufficient control over shape is the lack of appropriate scaffolds. The optimal scaffold used for engineering a cartilage construct with accurate designed shapes should possess at least three characteristics: good biocompatibility for cell seeding, ease of being processed into a specific shape, and sufficient mechanical strength for retaining the pre-designed shape. Polyglycolic acid (PGA) has proven to be one of the most successful scaffolds for cartilage regeneration [10- 12]. Cartilage engineered with the PGA scaffold has structure and composition similar to the native tissue, as demonstrated by histological analysis and cartilage specific matrices [13- 15]. However, the most widely used form of PGA material in cartilage engineering is unwoven fiber mesh, which is difficult to be initially prepared into a complicated 3D structure and would most likely fail to maintain its original architecture during subsequent *in vitro* chondrogenesis due to insufficient mechanical support [14, 16, 17].

To overcome these problems, two crucial issues should be addressed. First, the PGA-based scaffold should be prefabricated into the exact shape of human nose. Second, the mechanical strength of the above-mentioned scaffold should be further enhanced so that it can retain the pre-designed shape.

In order to meet these requirements, in the current study, a computer aided design and manufacturing (CAD/CAM) technique was employed to fabricate a set of negative molds, which was then used to press the PGA fibers into the pre-designed nose structure. Furthermore, the mechanical strength of the scaffold was enhanced by coating the PGA fibers with an optimized amount of PLA.

2. Materials and methods

2.1. Preparation of scaffolds with different PLA contents

10 mg of unwoven PGA fibers (provided by Dong Hua University, Shanghai, China) were compressed into a cylinder shape of 5mm in diameter and 2mm in thickness. A solution of 0.3 % PLA (Sigma, St. Louis, MO, USA) in dichloromethane was evenly dropped onto the PGA scaffold, dried in a 65 °C oven, and weighed. The PLA mass ratio was calculated according to the formula: PLA%= (final mass-original mass)/final mass×100%. The above procedures were repeated until the predetermined PLA mass ratios of 0%, 10%, 20%, 30%, 40% and 50% were achieved. The scaffolds were examined by SEM (Philips XL-30, Amsterdam, Netherlands) [18].

2.2. Biocompatibility evaluation of the scaffolds

Cell seeding: Chondrocytes were isolated from the articular cartilage of newborn swine (2-3weeks old) as previously described [19]. The harvested chondrocytes were adjusted to a final concentration of $50×10^6$ cells/mL, and a 100uL cell suspension was pipetted onto each scaffold. The cell-scaffold constructs were then incubated for 4h at 37°C with 95% humidity and 5% CO_2 to allow for complete adhesion of the cells to the scaffolds.

Cell adhesion: After 4 hours of incubation, the cell-scaffold constructs were gently transferred into a new 6-well plate. The remaining cells were collected and counted. The cell seeding efficiencies of the scaffolds with different PLA contents were calculated based on the formula: (total cell number- remaining cell number)/ total cell number×100% [14].

2.3. Mold fabrication by CAD/CAM

A patient's normal nose was scanned by CT to obtain the geometric data (Figure 3). These data were further processed by a CAD system to generate both positive and negative of the normal nose, and the resultant data were input into a CAM system (Spectrum 510, Z Corporation) for the fabrication of the resin models by 3D printing. The negative mold was composed of two parts: the anterior part and the posterior part. (Figure 4A)

2.4. Fabrication of nose shaped scaffold

Two hundred milligrams of unwoven PGA fibers were pressed using the negative mold for over 12 hours. A solution of 0.3 % PLA (Sigma, St. Louis, MO, USA) in dichloromethane was evenly dropped onto the PGA scaffold, dried in a 65 °C oven, weighed, and pressed again with the negative mold. This procedure was repeated until the final PLA mass ratio of 20% was reached. The edge of the scaffold was carefully trimmed according to the shape of the positive mold.

2.5. Statistical analysis

The differences of cell seeding efficiencies (n=6) among the six PLA content groups were analyzed using the Student's t-test. A p-value less than 0.05 was considered statistically significant.

3. Results

3.1. SEM observation of the scaffolds with different PLA contents

PLA/PGA scaffold compositions were visualized under SEM. (Figure 1) The pure PGA scaffold (0% PLA added) appeared as a smooth fiber mesh. In PGA scaffolds supplemented with 10% PLA, the PLA coating can be seen connecting some fibers, particularly at nodes where PGA fibers cross. In the 20% PLA embedded scaffold, most mesh nodes visualized were covered with PLA. 30% PLA scaffold had not only most mesh nodes embedded in PLA, but also the PLA coating was seen covering small portions of the mesh itself, minimally obstructing the porosity of the fiber network. In the 40% PLA embedded scaffold, most of the mesh porosity is obscured by a PLA. In the 50% PLA scaffold, the mesh is almost completely obscured by a PLA sheet.

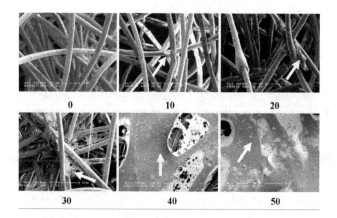

Figure 1. SEM examination. Scaffolds with different PLA contents (0%, 10%, 20%, 30%, 40% and 50%) show different pore structures. The white arrows indicate the coated PLA.

3.2. Evaluation of the biocompatibility of the scaffolds with different PLA contents

Cell seeding efficiencies were performed to evaluate the influence of PLA contents on cell compatibility of the scaffolds. The results showed that the increase in PLA content could lead to the reduction in the ability of the scaffolds to absorb the cell suspensions (Figure 2A). Quantitative analysis (Figure 2B) demonstrated that all the groups with PLA presented significantly lower cell seeding efficiencies compared to the group without PLA ($p<0.05$). If the acceptable cell adhesion rate is defined over 80%, these results indicate that 20% but not 30% is an acceptable PLA amount for preparing the scaffolds in terms of cell seeding efficiency.

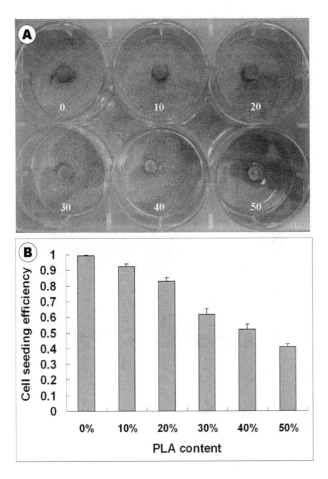

Figure 2. The influences of PLA contents on cell seeding efficiency. (A): Scaffolds with different PLA contents absorb different volumes of the cell suspension. (B): Cell seeding efficiencies decrease with increasing PLA contents in the scaffolds with significant decreases ($p<0.05$).

3.3. Mold preparation and fabrication of the nose-shaped scaffold

Because good biocompatibility could be achieved in the scaffold with 20% PLA, this formulation was further used for the fabrication of the human nose shaped scaffold. In order to prepare the scaffold into a shape of normal nose, a set of negative molds was produced according to image of the normal nose (Figure 3). The resulting nose-shaped scaffold (Figure 4C) achieved a precise shape compared to its positive mold (Figure 4B). These results indicate that the mold produced by CAD/CAM technology is allowed to accurately fabricate a scaffold into a nose shape.

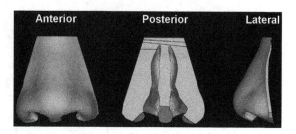

Figure 3. image of a patient's normal nose.

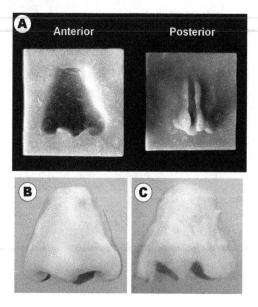

Figure 4. Mold preparation and the fabrication of the nose-shaped scaffolds. (A): The resin negative mold: anterior part and posterior part; (B): The resin positive mold; (C): the nose-shaped PLA/PGA scaffold.

4. Discussions

Despite the rapid progress in cartilage engineering, *in vitro* engineering of cartilage with a fine controlled 3D structure, such as human nose, remains a great challenge due to the lack of appropriate scaffolds. PGA has proven to be one of the most successful scaffolds for cartilage regeneration. However, for *in vitro* engineering of a cartilage with a precise shape, PGA unwoven fibers (the most widely used physical form) still have some drawbacks, such as the difficulties in controlling an accurate shape.

To achieve this, a negative mold corresponding to the desired shape is required. CAD/CAM, as a novel technique, has been widely used for the fabrication of anatomically accurate 3D models [20- 23]. Particularly, this method can accurately perform complicated manipulations of the original 3D data, including Boolean operations, mirror imaging, and scaling [24- 26]. CAD/CAM technique was therefore used in the current study for the production of the negative mold for a human nose. Using this mold, PGA fibers were able to be accurately prepared into the nose-shaped scaffold.

The mechanical strength of PGA scaffold alone is not sufficient for the shape maintenance, and thus PLA coating was used to strengthen its mechanical properties as reported [10, 11, 27]. However, a high amount of PLA in the scaffold would negatively affect cartilage formation because of poor cell compatibility [14]. Therefore, an appropriate PLA content in the scaffold is important for both shape maintenance and biocompatibility. In the current study, we evaluated the effects of six PLA contents on the scaffolds' biocompatibility. According to the current results, although the mechanical strength of the scaffolds increased with increasing PLA content, 20% is an acceptable PLA amount for preparing the scaffolds in terms of cell seeding efficiency.

Finally, aided by CAD/CAM technique, the PGA fibers were prepared into the accurate shape of a human nose. Furthermore, by coating with PLA, the scaffold could obtain sufficient mechanical strength to retain the original shape. These results may provide useful information for future nose reconstructions by *in vitro* engineered cartilage as well as for the engineering of other tissues with complicated 3D structures.

In summary, this study established a method to precisely engineer a PGA/PLA scaffold with the shape of human nose. In future studies, we will also investigate the fate of these scaffolds after cell seeding, especially subcutaneous implantation in an immunocompetent animal model.

Acknowledgements

This research was supported by National Natural Science Foundation of China (81101438 and 81201476).

Author details

Qiong Li, Lu Zhang*, Guangdong Zhou, Wei Liu and Yilin Cao

*Address all correspondence to: luzhangmd@gmail.com

Department of Plastic and Reconstructive Surgery, Shanghai th People's Hospital, Shanghai Jiao Tong University School of Medicine, Shanghai Key Laboratory of Tissue Engineering, Shanghai, P.R. China

References

[1] Bloom, J. D, Antunes, M. B, & Becker, D. G. Anatomy, physiology, and general concepts in nasal reconstruction. Facial Plast Surg Clin North Am (2011). , 19(1), 1-11.

[2] Immerman, S, White, W. M, & Constantinides, M. Cartilage grafting in nasal reconstruction. Facial Plast Surg Clin North Am (2011). , 19(1), 175-82.

[3] Romo, T. rd, Pearson JM. Nasal implants. Facial Plast Surg Clin North Am (2008). vi., 16(1), 123-32.

[4] Graham, B. S, Thiringer, J. K, & Barrett, T. L. Nasal tip ulceration from infection and extrusion of a nasal alloplastic implant. J Am Acad Dermatol (2001). Suppl):, 362-4.

[5] Langer, R, & Vacanti, J. P. Tissue engineering. Science (1993). , 260(5110), 920-6.

[6] Zhang, L. It is time to reconstruct human auricle more precisely and microinvasively. Plast Reconstr Surg (2010). e-156e.

[7] Zhang, L, & Spector, M. Tissue Engineering of Musculoskeletal Tissue. In: Pallua N, Suschek C, eds. Tissue Engineering: From Lab to Clinic:Springer,(2011).

[8] Cao, Y, Vacanti, J. P, Paige, K. T, Upton, J, & Vacanti, C. A. Transplantation of chondrocytes utilizing a polymer-cell construct to produce tissue-engineered cartilage in the shape of a human ear. Plast Reconstr Surg (1997). discussion 303-4., 100(2), 297-302.

[9] Kamil, S. H, Kojima, K, Vacanti, M. P, Bonassar, L. J, Vacanti, C. A, & Eavey, R. D. In vitro tissue engineering to generate a human-sized auricle and nasal tip. Laryngoscope (2003). , 113(1), 90-4.

[10] Cui, L, Wu, Y, Cen, L, Zhou, H, Yin, S, Liu, G, Liu, W, & Cao, Y. Repair of articular cartilage defect in non-weight bearing areas using adipose derived stem cells loaded polyglycolic acid mesh. Biomaterials (2009). , 30(14), 2683-93.

[11] Frenkel, S. R. Di Cesare PE. Scaffolds for articular cartilage repair. Ann Biomed Eng (2004). , 32(1), 26-34.

[12] Heath, C. A, & Magari, S. R. Mini-review: Mechanical factors affecting cartilage regeneration in vitro. Biotechnol Bioeng (1996). , 50(4), 430-7.

[13] Aufderheide, A. C, & Athanasiou, K. A. Comparison of scaffolds and culture conditions for tissue engineering of the knee meniscus. Tissue Eng (2005).

[14] Moran, J. M, Pazzano, D, & Bonassar, L. J. Characterization of polylactic acid-polyglycolic acid composites for cartilage tissue engineering. Tissue Eng (2003). , 9(1), 63-70.

[15] Yan, D, Zhou, G, Zhou, X, Liu, W, Zhang, W. J, Luo, X, Zhang, L, Jiang, T, Cui, L, & Cao, Y. The impact of low levels of collagen IX and pyridinoline on the mechanical properties of in vitro engineered cartilage. Biomaterials (2009). , 30(5), 814-21.

[16] Gunatillake, P. A, & Adhikari, R. Biodegradable synthetic polymers for tissue engineering. Eur Cell Mater (2003). discussion 16., 5, 1-16.

[17] Kim, B. S, & Mooney, D. J. Engineering smooth muscle tissue with a predefined structure. J Biomed Mater Res (1998). , 41(2), 322-32.

[18] Liu, Y, Zhang, L, Zhou, G, Li, Q, Liu, W, Yu, Z, Luo, X, Jiang, T, Zhang, W, & Cao, Y. In vitro engineering of human ear-shaped cartilage assisted with CAD/CAM technology. Biomaterials (2010). , 31(8), 2176-83.

[19] Zhang, L, & Spector, M. Comparison of three types of chondrocytes in collagen scaffolds for cartilage tissue engineering. Biomed Mater (2009).

[20] Bill, J. S, Reuther, J. F, Dittmann, W, Kubler, N, Meier, J. L, Pistner, H, & Wittenberg, G. Stereolithography in oral and maxillofacial operation planning. Int J Oral Maxillofac Surg (1995). Pt 2):98-103.

[21] Ciocca, L, Mingucci, R, Gassino, G, & Scotti, R. CAD/CAM ear model and virtual construction of the mold. J Prosthet Dent (2007). , 98(5), 339-43.

[22] Erickson, D. M, Chance, D, Schmitt, S, & Mathis, J. An opinion survey of reported benefits from the use of stereolithographic models. J Oral Maxillofac Surg (1999). , 57(9), 1040-3.

[23] Subburaj, K, Nair, C, Rajesh, S, Meshram, S. M, & Ravi, B. Rapid development of auricular prosthesis using CAD and rapid prototyping technologies. Int J Oral Maxillofac Surg (2007). , 36(10), 938-43.

[24] Al Mardini MErcoli C,Graser GN. A technique to produce a mirror-image wax pattern of an ear using rapid prototyping technology. J Prosthet Dent (2005). , 94(2), 195-8.

[25] Ciocca, L, & Scotti, R. CAD-CAM generated ear cast by means of a laser scanner and rapid prototyping machine. J Prosthet Dent (2004). , 92(6), 591-5.

[26] Karayazgan-saracoglu, B, Gunay, Y, & Atay, A. Fabrication of an auricular prosthesis using computed tomography and rapid prototyping technique. J Craniofac Surg (2009). , 20(4), 1169-72.

[27] Yang, S, Leong, K. F, Du, Z, & Chua, C. K. The design of scaffolds for use in tissue engineering. Part I. Traditional factors. Tissue Eng (2001). , 7(6), 679-89.

Chapter 7

Cartilage Tissue Engineering: The Role of Extracellular Matrix (ECM) and Novel Strategies

Zaira Y. García-Carvajal, David Garciadiego-Cázares,
Carmen Parra-Cid, Rocío Aguilar-Gaytán,
Cristina Velasquillo , Clemente Ibarra and
Javier S. Castro Carmona

Additional information is available at the end of the chapter

1. Introduction

Articular cartilage is a hyaline cartilage that consists primarily of extracellular matrix with a sparse population of cells, lacking blood vessels, lymphatic vessels and nerves. The only cell type within cartilage is the chondrocyte and has a low level of metabolic activity with little or no cell division and is the responsible for maintaining in a low-turnover state the unique composition and organization of the matrix that was determined during embryonic and postnatal development. The biological and mechanical properties of articular cartilage depend on the interactions between the chondrocytes and the matrix that maintain the tissue. Chondrocytes form the macromolecular framework of the tissue matrix from three classes of molecules: collagens, proteoglycans, and non-collagenous proteins and maintain the extracellular matrix (ECM) by low-turnover replacement of certain matrix proteins [1, 2].

Aggrecan and type II collagen are the most abundant proteins found within the ECM in the articular cartilage and they are linked together by a number of collagen-binding proteins including cartilage oligomeric matrix protein (COMP), chondroadherin and other minor collagens on their surface. Aggrecan is a large aggregating proteoglycan which is in association with hyaluronan (HA) and link protein (LP). These aggregates are responsible for the turgid and they provide the osmotic properties to resist compressive loads and retain water. Also contain a variety of small leucine-rich repeat proteoglycans (SLRPs) as decorin, biglycan, fibromodulin and lumican where they help maintain the integrity of the tissue and modulate its metabolism [3, 4].

2. Alteration in cartilage composition in Osteoarthritis (OA)

The chondrocyte is responsible for both the synthesis and the breakdown of the cartilaginous matrix but the mechanisms that control this balance are poorly understood [4]. The distribution of load across the joint is an important function of the articular cartilage for avoid excessive load affecting both cartilage and bone. It has been demonstrated that articular chondrocytes are able to respond to mechanical injury where biological stimuli such as cytokines and growth and differentiation factors contribute to structural changes in the surrounding cartilage matrix. It has been demonstrated that many non-mechanical and mechanical factors such as load clearly have a role in the initiation and propagation the processes of OA. The OA is the most common joint disease allowing dysfunction and pain. The OA is characterized by changes in chondrocyte metabolism that leads to elevated production of proteolytic enzymes, cartilage damage and loss of joint function. It have been described several mechanisms that can lead to OA, among of these mechanisms are mechanicals, bone changes and changes in the cartilage extracellular matrix [5, 6]

Aging, cartilage senescence and reactive oxygen species (ROS) are normal changes in the musculoskeletal system that contribute to the development of OA, but the mechanisms are poorly understood [5]. Inflammation is considered as a very early event in OA perhaps induced by joint trauma affecting chondrocytes in the cartilage and synovial cells (fibroblasts and macrophages) to produce cytokines as interleukin-1-beta (IL-1β) and tumoral necrosis factor-alpha (TNF-α), and other signaling molecules as proteoglycans to switch to or increase catabolic processes [6]. Obesity has been described as a risk factor for OA by increased mechanical load factors and degenerative knee pain. The mechanisms between obesity and OA are not completly understood but, it has been found the release of fat molecules that can affect the processes in the joint, including adipokines as visfatin and leptin, perhaps affecting the inflammatory response [7, 9]. Malalignment of the knee joint plays an important role in the development of early osteoarthritis changing the center of pressure of articular cartilage and subchondral bone. Varus or valgus malalignment of the lower extremity results in an abnormal load distribution across the medial and lateral tibiofemoral compartment and being increased in patients with knee osteoarthritis and is increased in patients with overweight. However, studies examining the relationship between malalignment and early knee osteoarthritis have produced conflicting results. The association between malalignment and OA changes is based on radiographic changes mainly and different multicenter OA studies [10-12]. Meniscus is an important tissue in the system of the knee. It is function is the load transmission and absortion shock. Complete or partial loss of meniscal tissue alters the biomechanical and biological of the knee joint modifying the pattern of load distribution and the instability of the knee. Meniscal narrowing, cartilage loss and chondral lesions increase the risk of secondary OA with cartilage degeneration. This secondary OA is associated to chondral damage, ligamentous instability, and malalignment with reduction in the shock absorption capacity of the knee [13-15]. Extrusion has been associated with articular changes according to their depth into partial-thickness and full-thickens defects. Partial-thickness lesions are considered less symptomatic with little evidence of progression on osteoarthritis. Full-thickness chondral and osteochondral lesions frequently cause symptoms, and they are considered to predispose to premature osteoarthritis [16]. Osteochondritis dissecans studies have demonstrated knee joint dysfunction and high prevalence of osteoarthritic change after fragment removal and all the studies take in account the limitation of a small defect size from 1.5 to 4.0 cm^2 as well the zone and the location of the defect in the cartilage [17, 18]. The anterior cruciate ligament (ACL) is the knee ligament most common disrupted. ACL lesion frequently is associated to other ligamentous structures like, menisci, the articular cartilage or subchondral plate [19, 20].

3. Articular cartilage homeostasis

Articular cartilage is composed of four distinct regions and they differ in their collagen fibril orientation: (a) the superficial or tangential zone (200 μm), (b) the middle or transitional zone, (c) the deep or radial zone and (d) the calcified cartilage zone. The superficial zone is composed of thin collagen fibrils in tangential array parallel to surface with a high concentration of decorin and lubricin and a low concentration of aggrecan. The middle zone is composed thicker collagen fibrils more random organized. The deep zone is composed the collagen bundles thickest and arranged in a radial fashion, orthogonal to the surface, and the calcified cartilage zone, located above subchondral bone and the tidemark that persists after growth plate closure and is composed of matrix vesicles, vascularization and innervation from the subchondral bone. The collagen type in the calcified zone surrounding the cells is type X as in the hypertrofic zone of the growth plate [21, 22], [23]. From the superficial to the deep zone, cell density progressively decreases. The chondrocytes in the superficial zone are small and flattened. The chondrocytes in the middle zone are rounded, and the deep zone chondrocytes are grouped in columns or clusters and they are larger and express markers of the hypertrophy as well. Differences in expression of zonal subpopulations may determine the zonal differences in matrix composition and in the mechanical environment [24, 25].

Chondrocytes live at low oxygen tension within the cartilage matrix, ranging from 10% at the surface to less than 1% in the deep zones. *In vitro*, chondrocytes adapt to low oxygen tensions by up-regulating hypoxia-inducible factor-1-alpha (HIF-1α), which stimulate expression of glucose transport via constitutive glucose transporter proteins (GLUTs) and angiogenic factors such as vascular endothelial growth factor (VEGF) as well as a number of genes associated with cartilage anabolism and chondrocyte differentiation [26, 27].

It is no clear how chondrocytes maintain their ECM under normal conditions since they lack access to the vascular system but gene expression and protein synthesis may be activated by injury. The aging may affect the properties of normal cartilage by altering the content, composition and structural organization of collagen and proteoglycans. The normal function of the articular cartilage within the joint is to be elastic and have high tensile strength and these properties depend on the extracellular matrix [28]. The chondrocytes produce, in appropriate amounts, this ECM that consist of structural macromolecules of type II collagen fibers, proteoglycans, non-collagenous proteins and glycoproteins, organized into a highly ordered molecular framework. The collagen matrix gives cartilage its form and tensile strength. Proteoglycans and non-collagenous proteins bind to the collagenous network and help to stabilize the matrix framework and bind the chondrocytes to the macromolecules of the network. The matrix protects the cells from injury due to normal use of the joint, determines the types and concentrations of molecules that reach the cells and helps to maintain the chondrocyte phenotype [29, 30].

The ECM surrounding the chondrocytes has been divided into zones depending on their distance from the cell. The pericellular matrix is localized immediately around the cell, the territorial matrix is next to pericellular matrix and the most distance is the interterritorial matrix. Each matrix zone is characterized by different types of collagens as shown in figure 1.

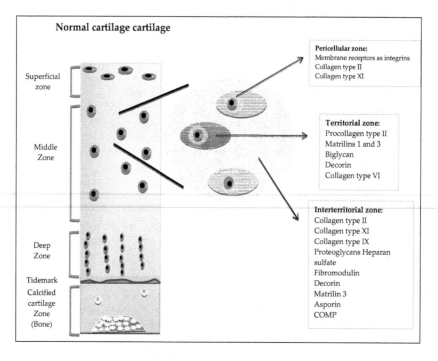

Figure 1. The organization of normal articular cartilage. The organization of chondrocytes is divided in superficial, middle or transitional, deep or radial and calcified cartilage zones with a boundary or tidemark between the first three zones and the calcified zone. The extracellular matrix is divided depending the distance from the chondrocytes. The pericellular zone is the matrix surrounding immediately the chondrocytes. The territorial zone is the next to pericellular zone and the interterritorial zone is the most distant. Every zone has specific characteristics related with the shape of the chondrocyte as well the activity and the expression of different molecules by the cell.

The pericellular matrix is a region surrounding chondrocytes in the articular cartilage where diverse molecules as growth factors have interaction with the receptors expressed on the membrane cell of chondrocyte. This region is rich in proteoglycans as aggrecan, hyaluronan and decorin. Type II, VI and IX are collagen most concentrated in the pericellular network of thin fibrils as fibronectin. Type VI collagen forms part of the matrix immediately surrounding the chondrocytes and may help them to attach to the macromolecular framework of the matrix. This pericellular matrix enclosed cells has been termed chondron. The territorial zone contains type VI collagen microfibrils but little or no fibrillar collagen. The interterritorial cartilage matrix is composed of a collagen type II, type XI collagen and type IX collagen integrated in the fibril surface with the non-collagen domain, permitting association with other matrix components and retention of proteoglycans. These collagens give to the cartilage form, tensile stiffness and strength [31-33].

Cartilage contains a variety of proteoglycans that are essential for its normal function. These include aggrecan, decorin, biglycan, fibromodulin and lumican each proteoglycan has several functions determined. The proteoglycans are very important for protecting the collagen network. Other non-collagen molecules as the matrilins and cartilage oligomeric protein (COMP) are also present in the matrix. COMP acts as a catalyst in collagen fibrillogenesis, and interactions between type IX collagen and COMP or matrilin-3 are essential for proper formation and maintenance of the articular cartilage matrix. Perlecan enhances fibril formation, and collagen VI microfibrils connect to collagen II and aggrecan via complexes of matrilin-1 and biglycan or decorin [34].

Throughout life, the cartilage undergoes continual internal remodeling and the chondrocytes replace matrix macromolecules lost through degradation. Therefore normal matrix turnover depends on the ability of chondrocytes to detect alterations in the macromolecular composition and organization of the matrix, including the presence of degraded molecules, and to respond by synthesizing appropriate types and amounts of new molecules. In addition, the matrix acts as a signal transducer for the cells. Loading of the tissue due to use of the joint creates mechanical, electrical, and physicochemical signals that help to direct the synthetic and degradative activity of chondrocytes [22, 35].

4. Extracellular matrix and cell signaling

Chondrocytes respond to the mechanical and biochemical changes in ECM through signaling events by various cell surface growth factor receptors and adhesion molecules. ECM proteins can determine the cell behavior, polarity, migration, differentiation, proliferation and survival by communicating with the intracellular cytoskeleton and transmission of growth factor signals. Integrins and proteoglycans are the major ECM adhesion receptors, which cooperate in signaling events, determining the signaling events, and thus the cell function [36].

Integrins are heterodimeric transmembrane receptors formed of eighteen α subunits and eight β subunits and they are non-covalently assembled into 24 combinations. The integrin dimers bind to different ECM molecules with overlapping binding affinities determining expression patterns and the downstream signaling events in the cell. Integrins respond specifically to the molecular composition and physical properties of the ECM and integrate both mechanical and chemical signals through direct association with the cytoskeleton. Integrins recognize and bind to the Arg-Gly-Asp (RGD) motif that they are attachment sites for integrin mediated cell adhesion. It has been demonstrated that high density of

RGD motifs allows a precise spatial distribution pattern of integrins for specific cellular response among ligand molecules [36, 37].

Integrins can activate several signaling pathways independently and frequently they act synergistically with other growth factor receptors as insulin receptor, type 1 insulin-like growth factor receptor, VEGF receptor, TGF-b receptor, platelet-derived growth factor-b (PDGF-b) receptor and epidermal growth factor (EGF) receptor [37,38].

4.1. Role of proteoglycans in signal regulation

The heparan sulfate proteoglycans (HSPGs) contribute to the organization of the matrix by binding to the many core matrix molecules via HS chains as laminin, fibronectin and collagen. The chondroitin sulphate proteoglycans (CSPGs) as aggrecan, versican, brevican and the small, leucine-rich proteoglycans such as decorin and biglycan also bind to and regulate a number of growth factors, such as members of the TGF family. The hyaluronic acid is a glycosamino-glycan synthesized on the cell surface and is responsible for the gel-like consistency of cartilage by its hydroscopic properties [36, 39].

4.2. Remodelation and degradation of ECM

During normal or pathologic physiology of the cartilage, the ECM must be remodeling and degraded to allow the chondrocytes for processing and deposition of new matrix by specific proteases. There are two well-known families of proteases that are involved in the biology of the ECM, the matrix metalloproteinase (MMP) and the desintegrins and metalloproteinases with thrombospondin motif (ADAMTS) families. The MMP-13 is involved in the cleavage of fibromodulin and type IX collagen and is present and active in the pathological process of cartilage as OA and rheumatoid arthritis. The aggrecanases family's ADAMTS-4 and ADAMTS-5 play an important role in cartilage damage during early OA which cleavage the glycosaminoglycans chains that are the key contributors to the maintenance of the charge density, the osmotic environment and water retain important characteristics of the mechanical properties of the cartilage [40, 41].

5. Alterations of the ECM in the skeletal tissue: Injuries and pathologies

The extracellular matrix has structural and functional relevance, it's a highly organized and assembled macromolecular structure, also provide cellular adhesion environments, activation and inactivation of growth factors and regulatory cytokines. The proteolytic processing of ECM components, results in the production of fragments with biological effects on migration, proliferation and cellular organization.

When any component of the ECM has a disorder, could generate chondrodysplasia, it means alterations in the development and growth of cartilage. Chondrodysplasias are caused by various mutations in genes involved in cartilage development and finally in the formation and growth of the long bones. These mutations also often alter the formation of other tissues.

Achondrogenesis type II, is a chondrodysplasia classified as collagenopathy type II. In this family are located several chondrodysplasia caused by mutations in the gene for collagen II, which is the most abundant protein in cartilage [42]. These dysplasias are, achondrogenesis type II, hypochondrogenesis, congenital espondiloepiphysial dysplasia and Kniest dysplasia, among others. Collagen II is a homotrimer (three identical chains encoded by the COL2A1 gene located on chromosome 12. This collagen is mainly found in the hyaline cartilage and vitreous humor, so its deficiency is associated with abnormalities of the spine, of the epiphysis and eye problems. Despite their differences these dysplasias share clinical and radiological manifestations, so the axial skeleton is affected more than the limbs, cleft palate, myopia and retinal degeneration [43].

Furthermore, other disorders of matrix components such as collagen IX and XI, which interact with the collagen II to form supramolecular structures, are closely related phenomena.

It is found that the Osteogenesis Imperfecta (OI) is caused by molecular defects of collagen type I[44] and metaphyseal chondrodysplasia Schmid type is caused by errors in collagen type X biosynthesis [45], the latter is characterized by alterations in vertebrae and in the metaphysis of long bones, also show reduction of the area of reserve cartilage in growth plate and in the articular cartilage, alters the contents of bone and there is an atypical distribution of the matrix components of the growth plate.

The cartilage oligomeric matrix protein (COMP) is a member trombospondins family, and its alteration causes pseudoachondroplasia, this disorder shows short limbs and lax ligaments [46], the growth plate is shorter and the area of hypertrophic cartilage is reduced.

Cartilage needs molecular signals for development and maintenance, such as growth factors, which in many cases are regulating the synthesis of the ECM, and may be found active or latent in the extracellular matrix. Bone morphogenetic proteins (BMPs), transforming growth factor beta (TGF-β), growth and differentiation factor 5 (GDF-5), are signals related to the development and growth of cartilage, alterations in these molecules cause some malformations, such as the brachypodism (short limbs) [47].

Cartilage matrix is rich in sulfated proteoglycans and the gene encoding for sulfate transporter called DTDST (Dystrophic Dysplasia Sulfate Transporter) in patients with dystrophic dysplasia was found mutations in this gene, and shown to be deficient cartilage sulfating [48].

Campomelic dysplasia is a rare disease associated with XY individuals who possess varying degrees of sex reversal. SOX-9 is a transcription factor structurally related to the gene SRY (sex-determining region Y) required for testicular development. However, SOX-9 also directly regulates the gene for type II collagen, the main molecule of the cartilage matrix and therefore of chondrocyte differentiation [49, 50, 51].

The inactivation of the gene coding for the mouse gelatinase B, defined the mechanism that controls the final step of the chondrocyte maturation [52]. Gelatinase B is an enzyme present in the extracellular matrix of cartilage and its activity is related to the control of apoptosis of hypertrophic chondrocytes and the vascular tissue. This study hypothesized the existence of chondroclast, these cells of myeloid origin express gelatinase-B and are located in the cartilage/bone region and resorb cartilage matrix.

Based on the above is to emphasize the importance of the extracellular matrix as a modulator of cellular differentiation of chondrocytes, the extracellular components correlate with the differentiation state. That is, collagen I is present at early stages of differentiation and maturation, in mesenchyme and perichondrium; collagen II is on mature cartilage and collagen X is exclusive of hypertrophic cartilage also collagen type I are expressed in terminal stages of chondrocytes [53].

The ECM not only serves as a binder that gives form to tissues in addition to their structural role has physiological functions. The chondrocytes are in the array a series of signals that allows them to gain some cell shape and organization of the cytoskeletal network. Cell morphology that can modulate many physiological functions such as proliferation, differentiation, cell death and gene expression. This transmembrane receptor-mediated would be able to receive the extracellular signal from the ECM and transduce the signal into the cell, triggering a response by the chondrocyte differentiation [54].

Integrins are transmembrane receptor consisting of one α subunit and a β, are only functional to form the α-β heterodimer on the cell membrane. $\beta 1$ family of integrins are major receptors of ECM molecules and have the ability to allow cell adhesion and simultaneously issuing an intracellular signal to which the cell responds in different ways, as also interact with integrins the cytoskeleton and molecules involved in signal transduction.

It has been shown that integrins interaction with extracellular matrix molecules affects cytoskeleton organization, proliferation, differentiation and gene expression in fibroblasts and epithelial cells.

In addition we have studied the survival and differentiation of chondrocytes, including the deposit in the interstitial matrix of collagen type X could be mediated by integrins [55]. Inhibition of integrin b1 subunit with a neutralizing antibody blocks the deposition of collagen X in the interstitial matrix and growth of the breastbone is decreased. Moreover, the chondrocytes are significantly smaller, show a disorganization of the actin cytoskeleton and show increased apoptosis.

There is also evidence that blocking the $\beta 1$ subunit of integrins in an in vitro model of differentiation of cartilage inhibits cartilage nodule formation and the synthesis of collagen type II [56].

However, the study of the role of these receptors in the process of chondrocyte differentiation is not yet well established, but it would be of significant importance in determining the relationship of the extracellular matrix to the chondrocyte.

5.1. The extracellular matrix and chondrocyte differentiation in osteoarthritis

Articular cartilage mineralization frequently accompanies and complicates osteoarthritis and aging. Several works has demonstrated that certain features of growth cartilage development are shared in degenerative cartilage. These include chondrocyte proliferation, hypertrophy, matrix mineralization and apoptosis. Development of growth plate is regulated by growth factors signaling and cellular interactions with the extracellular matrix (ECM). Parathyroid hormone related protein (PthrP) and Indian Hedgehog (Ihh) are central mediators of endo-chondral development; PthrP is abundant in synovial fluid of osteoarthritic patient but Ihh expression is diminish in OA cartilage, Fgf-18 is a regulator of chondrocyte proliferation and its intra-synovial application in OA rat results in cartilage generation. Also, Wnt signaling plays an important role in chondrocyte differentiation in growth plate, Wnt-5a promotes chondrocyte prehypertrophy and inhibits chondrocyte hypertrophy unlike Wnt-4 that induces chondrocyte hypertrophy and increases its expression in early stage of osteoarthritis. On the other hand, is pronounced imbalance of cartilage matrix turnover in osteoarthritic cartilage, and results in mayor deposition of collagen type I and X, reduced expression of collagen type II. Thus, the rate of chondrocyte hypertrophy is higher on growth plate and OA articular cartilage than healthy articular cartilage, it recap the signaling in cartilage growth plate. But, although articular and growth plate cartilages share several features, there are one important difference, the rate of cartilage hypertrophy. What is the signal that makes the difference? In the ECM we could find some elements to answer this question.

5.1.1. Alterations in the extracellular matrix of articular cartilage during OA

Traditionally it has been thought that osteoarthritis is a disease of wear or tears consequence of articular cartilage due to aging or following injury. The limited regenerative capacity of cartilage cannot reverse its destruction, it is sometimes triggered by an inflammatory response from the synovial, inflammation occurs when the condition is called osteoarthritis [57]. Until recent years genetic mutations were excluded as a risk factor or predisposition to osteoarthritis. The first genes identified to OA encode components of the extracellular matrix, such as Collagen COL2A1, COL9A2 and COL11A2, which were studied in transgenic mouse models [58]. It has been found that the substitution of glycine destabilizes the triple helix structure of collagen type II making it more susceptible to degradation by MMP-13 [59]. Other ECM molecules related to OA are ADAMTS-4 and ADAMTS-5 enzymes which degrade aggrecan, the most abundant proteoglycan in articular cartilage [60]. When aggrecan is degraded, the collagen II is exposed to the DDR-2 enzyme which is able to degrade it [61]. The alteration of the ECM of articular cartilage in the first instance causes cell proliferation and the formation of fibrous tissue that forms a scar in response to injury, there are produced growth factors such as TGF-β could promote chondrocyte hypertrophy, so that recapitulates OA cartilage differ-entiation mechanisms of the growth plate to form ultimately bone nodules at the edges of articular cartilage called osteophytes [62]. Clearly the importance of ECM in the differentiation of articular cartilage, but there are various growth factors and transcription factors that regulate the maturation and proliferation of chondrocytes in articular cartilage and cartilage growth plate, which also control the expression of many of the components of the ECM, and also direct the skeletal morphogenesis. Genes has recently been determined as Smad-3, Dkk, Wnt4, Mig-6 etc [63- 66], OA generated in murine models, these molecules regulate different cellular processes such as cell proliferation, cell differentiation, cell death, degradation and synthesis of ECM. We can group the molecules according to the governing process: Chondro-genesis, Proliferation, Differentiation and Cell Death. Many of these molecules can be good genetic markers of predisposition to OA, and are fundamental to how to design a strategy for articular cartilage repair.

5.1.2. Differentiation of articular cartilage chondrocyte

Although exists different types of cartilage, they are very similar but have different functions. Articular cartilage and cartilage growth plate are good examples. In general, the molecular mechanisms of chondrocyte differentiation in both cartilages are equivalent. However, for the function of synovial joints is essential that chondrocytes maintenance in prehypertrophic state differentiation, while the longitudinal growth of bone depends on the proliferation and differentiation of chondrocytes in the growth plate to the hypertrophy and bone formation [67, 68]. We can even talk about a model that relates the structure and function of cartilage based on histological and functional differences of both cartilages. Both in the cartilage growth plate and in articular cartilage chondrocytes can be found at various stages of differentiation, but the organization and activity of chondrocytes differ in each stage of both cartilage.

In the growth plate chondrocytes reserves represent an immature state and are organized in tiny rows of small round cells, embedded in an abundant extracellular matrix rich in collagen type II and aggrecan, proliferating chondrocytes are stacked as "coins" several rows forming compact occupying a large area of the growth plate, the first rows are more proliferation activity than the rows deep; prehypertrofic chondrocytes (mature) are larger cells that have exited the cell cycle and express Ihh, a key molecule in cartilage differentiation, these cells secrete and accumulate a large amount of carbohydrates and finally the hypertrophic chondrocytes are cells of highest volume and high alkaline phosphatase activity, the ECM is mainly composed of collagen type X and begins to calcify, some cells degenerate and die by apoptosis leaving the spaces occupied to consolidate osteoblasts and bone tissue. This process is known as endochondral ossification which regulates the growth of bone in terms of cartilage differentiation. It is noteworthy that an important signaling center in this process is the perichondrium, which are very small and flattened cells surrounding the cartilage and expressed PTHrP [69] and Fgf-18 [70], which respectively induce and inhibit the proliferation of chondrocytes, the receiver PPR and PTHrP [71] is expressed in the upper rows, whereas the Fgf-18 receptor and FGF-R3 is found in the deeper cell layers of proliferating chondrocytes. Patch is Ihh receptor and is expressed in the perichondrium, so that Ihh induces the expression of PTHrP and this in turn induces proliferation and expression of Ihh in the growth plate. This regulatory loop promotes the longitudinal growth of the mold of cartilage, but it is necessary that the mold is rigid. For this, the FGF18 inhibits the proliferation of cartilage to regulate expression of Ihh and this result in the differentiation of chondrocyte hypertrophy up. This signaling cascade also occurs during the formation of joint cartilage, where bone formation is more limited as in the secondary ossification centers.

Articular cartilage has apparently different stages of differentiation of chondrocytes, only that which corresponds to the resting chondrocytes have important differences in the composition of the ECM, as the presence of lubricin, the Collagen type IIa the aggrecan, CD44, ASC, [72, 73] these cells are most abundant in the articular cartilage cells for proliferation area are not organized in rows and have very low proliferation rate, making them more similar to the prehypertrophic cartilage, as the rate of is very slow maturation, hypertrophic chondrocytes make up a small area of just one or two cell lines the border between cartilage and bone, known as "water mark" (tide mark).

5.2. Endochondral ossification during skeletal development and OA

The joints that separate from each other skeletal elements serve as important signaling centers during skeletal development, and regulate the proliferation and maturation of chondrocytes. It is well known that chondrocyte maturation is crucial for endochondral ossification and to define the final size of each skeletal element. In the end, the processes of the formation of joints and cartilage differentiation of skeletal elements are strongly related. The limb skeletal elements are formed by endochondral ossification, the process begins with the aggregation of mesenchymal cells that form the pre-cartilaginous condensation, this condensation increases the proliferation of chondrocytes and forms a "bar" initial cartilage [74]. It has been proposed that the first step for the formation of the joint is that it inhibits differentiation of prehypertrofic chondrocytes in cells located in the region of the joint prospecting, outside the influence of signals that promote maturation of the cartilage, while neighboring cells continue their differentiation process to form bone hypertrophy and subsequently by endochondral ossification, so contributing to the formation of adjacent skeletal elements [75]. Cells suspected joint region form the interzone, characterized by a highly packed region of flattened cells, these cells produce other types of collagen and collagen type I and III, unlike chondrocytes that produce collagen type II. The interzone also expressed molecules such as Wnt-9a [76] and Bmp antagonists like noggin [77], which remain the property of these cells not chondrogenic. Some cell adhesion molecules such as integrin α5β1 also regulate the formation of joints by controlling the differentiation of chondrocytes [78], whereas other signaling molecules that are expressed in the interzone as Wnt-4, Fgf-18, Gdf (5, 6 and 7) and several members of the Bmp, promote growth and differentiation of adjacent cartilaginous elements [79]. It is likely that different cell types present in a mature synovial joint, including synovial cells, articular chondrocytes and permanent joint capsule cells originate in the interzone. Permanent articular chondrocytes originating from the interzone, are very similar to chondrocytes in the growth plate, and although both cell types are hyaline cartilage and functions have important differences. The most important difference is that articular chondrocytes decrease its maturation toward hypertrophy of chondrocytes unlike the growth plate which we observed a wide region of hypertrophic chondrocytes, as this process allows for the ossification and growth of long bones. Hypertrophic chondrocytes are the highest volume and produce a very specific extracellular matrix rich in collagen type X. The hypertrophy of chondrocytes is followed by apoptosis, the invasion of blood vessels, osteoclasts and other mesenchymal cells from the perichondrium and production of bone matrix. Therefore, the size and fine structure of the long bones depends on the coordinated regulation of proliferation, maturation and hypertrophy of chondrocytes in response to many extracellular signals. The protein Indian hedgehog (Ihh) and peptide related to Thyroid Hormone (PTHrP) play a critical role in these processes, Ihh is produced by prehypertrophic chondrocytes and induces the expression of PTHrP in the perichondrium which in turn regulates the rate of chondrocytes which exit the cell cycle and continue to hypertrophy [80]. Ihh also stimulates proliferation of chondrocytes and controls the differentiation of mesenchymal cells into osteoblasts in the collar bone. Thus, when the chondrocytes stop expressing Ihh activates the expression of Runx-2 and Runx-3 [81], some transcription factors required for hypertrophy of chondrocytes and differentiation of osteoblasts. On the contrary, in particular FGF-18 [82] expressed in the perichondrium and through its receptor Fgf-R3 expressed in cartilage prehypertrofic cartilage negatively regulates cell proliferation and promotes the hypertrophy of chondrocytes, the constitutive activation of FGFR3 results in dwarfism [83] and may inhibit the formation of joints, this confirms the idea that proliferating chondrocytes may have two possible destinations, become pre-articular chondrocytes or prehypertrophic chondrocytes.

5.3. Control of chondrocyte differentiation and two destinations, Ihh vs Wnt signaling and its role in OA

During the formation of the skeleton some chondrocytes are involved in the growth of long bones and ossification. At this early stage, the GDF-5 signaling is essential for the formation of joints and articular cartilage [84, 85], its expression is delimited in the interzone and begins just before forming the joints, on the other hand, the Bmp-7 is important for the chondrocyte maturation and bone formation and is expressed in the perichondrium of the skeletal elements in formation and growth [86], but not expressed in the perichondrium of the developing cartilage. Although the induction of the joint is initiated by the expression of Wnt-9a in the interzone and the interzone chondrocytes lose their phenotype [76], GDF-5 signaling is essential for the joint and articular cartilage formation. Ihh is another important molecule for skeletal development, Ihh inhibits Wnt-9a expression and is maintained in skeletal growth and endochondral ossification, as when it reaches a certain size decreases the expression of Ihh and thereby activates the expression of Wnt patway induces hypertrophy of chondrocytes and bone formation [87]. It is noteworthy that during the OA Wnt signaling is overactivated [65] and GDF-5 is down-regulated, which suggests a recapitulation of endochondral ossification during OA. Furthermore, when the receptor Bmp-RIA is inactivated in mouse generated phenotypes similar to human osteoarthritis and when activated the Wnt pathway by blocking antagonist Dkk [64], reverse the process of articular cartilage destruction and endochondral ossification, this suggests that these pathways permit the maintenance of adult articular cartilage.

5.4. Proliferation, hypertrophy and cell death are activated during OA

Not only in the embryonic stages imbalance of proliferative signals and bring important consequences hypertrophy in articular cartilage, osteoarthritis is a striking example of this imbalance of signals. There are animal models that recapitulate this degenerative joint disease, as in the case of the mutant mice of Smad-3 [63], a molecule that transduces the TGF-β signal. Molecular analysis of these mice shows ectopic expression of type X collagen in the articular cartilage and increased hypertrophy of chondrocytes; this shows the TGF-β as an inhibitor of differentiation of articular chondrocytes. Similarly, the cancellation of Mig-6 in mice results in early degeneration of joints [66], as evidenced by degradation of articular cartilage, fibrous tissue formation and growth of osteophytes. It is well known that articular cartilage injuries may result in osteoarthritis, fibrous tissue formation is an immediate healing response to a traumatic injury, and the healing is often promoted by TGF-β, which in turn could induce osteophyte formation that recapitulates chondrogenesis and endochondral ossification in adult articular cartilage.

5.5. Why not articular cartilage regenerate

During development are constantly chondrocytes proliferation and differentiation, thus skeletal elements grow in length and ossify, as mentioned earlier, articular cartilage chondro-cytes have a low rate of proliferation and differentiation, this makes them different and allows articular cartilage is kept almost throughout life. What keeps the ever-growing cartilage during development is the molecular signals that modulate the rate of growth and differentiation, these signals are regulated by the perichondrium. The perichondrium has progenitor cells that are very useful for cartilage repair, its similar to bone, the periosteum is important for bone repair, such as fractures. While the perichondrium is maintained until adult stages, the perichondrium is disappearing from the stage young individuals, which is why the low capacity of regeneration of cartilage [88].

6. Current methods for cartilage tissue engineering and future perspectives

6.1. Autologous chondrocytes for tissue regeneration

The hyaline articular cartilage is a highly specialized tissue and its main function is to protect the bone from friction in the joints [89, 90], once articular cartilage is damaged their ability to self-repair and regeneration is limited as mentioned above. Cartilage injuries are mainly associated with anterior cruciate ligament, patellar dislocation, followed by a meniscectomy [91]. Osteochondral lesions of the knee are determined mainly by arthroscopic knee surgery [92, 93], which is seen mainly in traumatic injuries, together with abnormal stresses on the knee.

To determine the treatment for the repair and regeneration of articular cartilage injury, have developed different techniques, the techniques described are focused on the repair, recon-struction or regeneration of tissue. The repair methods (drilling or microfracture) support the formation of new tissue fibrocartilaginous [94, 95] while the reconstructive method seeks to fill the defect with allografts (OATS) combining with miniarthrotomy arthroscopy. And finally the regenerative methods that rely on bioengineering techniques to develop a hyaline cartilage tissue graft or autologous chondrocyte cell matrices (Table1).

Ref.	Method	Technique	Results
[96]	Drilling with lavage and debridement	Removal of osteophytes and knee abrasion	
[97]		Perform subchondral drilling of the lamina	Tissue repair and pain relief
[98]		Elimination of subchondral lamina	Significant symptomatic improvement in 75% of patients
[99, 100]	Microfracture	Perforation of the subchondral lamina by arthroscopy, it promotes the release of mesenchymal cells in the lesion, forming a plug of tissue	Avoids necrosis associated with the use of the drill and preserves the subchondral surface. The results observed in the medium term, mainly in young patients, about 20% of patients do not reach after five years.
[101-104]	Chondrogenesis induced stimulation of bone marrow (AMIC)	Followed by a micro abrasion bill and placing a collagen scaffold on the defect, inducing the formation of fibrocartilage by migrating mesenchymal cells and the expression of cytokines and tissue repair	Stimulation of bone marrow has limited mechanical strength and may even degrade the cartilage is repaired with fibrous tissue or fibrocartilage so that there is tissue degeneration.
[105-107]	Mosaicplasty and transplant osteochondral allograft	Is based on obtaining osteochondral cylinder obtained from areas of low load from the distal femur, which are grafted into the defect	The results are limited in large lesions due to donor site morbidity and healing of the seams in the recipient
[108-110]	Autologous chondrocyte implantation	1st Generation: In this technique, cartilage cells are injected under a cover of periosteum is sutured into the defect. 2nd. Generation: is replaced cover membrane or periosteum biomaterials, which can have different components	It has been reported good results in most patients after 10-20 years after implantation. In the second generation transplants with areas of fibrocartilage, possibly because of low cell density and lack of proliferative capacity. This technique replaces healthy cartilage to regularize the defect.
[111]	Autologous chondrocyte implantation induces extracellular matrix	3rd. Generation: In this technique, autologous chondrocytes cultured on a three-dimensional artificial scaffold	Has been used in the past two decades, with this type of membranes hypertrophy is reduced by 5%, after 3 to 6 months membrane is reabsorbed.

Table 1. Cartilage repair techniques

Each of these procedures is associated with improvement of these techniques with the use of biomaterials or with the use of growth factors. In the autologous chondrocyte implantation of the second generation is required arthrotomy so this technique becomes more complicated. In order to facilitate and improve the technique and quality of the tissue repair, has developed a method which has proved more effective and easy to implement in the knee joint [112, 113] develop and autologous chondrocyte implantation induced extracellular matrix of the third generation.

6.2. Description of the technique of autologous chondrocyte implantation induced extracellular matrix (third generation).

6.2.1. Obtaining the tissue

This technique is mainly based on the autologous cultured chondrocytes on a biocompatible three-dimensional scaffold which is subsequently implanted into the defect. As in the technique of autologous chondrocyte implantation of the second generation, it requires a prior arthroscopic surgery where a piece of cartilage obtained from a zone of no load of the knee joint (intercondylar notch or the lateral edge of the trochlea) after obtaining the sample fragment is processed to obtain chondrocytes in culture.

6.2.2. Implant preparation

Cartilage fragments are disintegrated mechanically to obtain smallest fragment, is performed subsequent enzymatic digestion to release trapped chondrocytes in the matrix of collagen. Expansion of chondrocytes was performed in 8 weeks. Days before implantation chondrocytes are seeded on a scaffold or membrane [112] Rich in collagen, which is considered a three-dimensional extracellular biomaterial consists mainly of collagen I and III, the scaffold contains glycosaminoglycans, proteoglycans and glycoproteins [111, 114, 115] cells are capable of synthesizing a typical matrix of chondrocytes facilitating cell adhesion and influence the morphology, migration and differentiation of cells.

6.3. Advantages of autologous chondrocyte transplantation induced extracellular matrix (third generation) on the autologous chondrocyte implantation (second generation)

The main advantages of autologous chondrocyte transplantation induced extracellular matrix (third generation) is that no cell loss is not presented hypertrophic tissue growth, requiring only a second incision is a safe procedure for treatment of injuries symptomatic articular cartilage surgery facilitates reducing the operating time and the need for open surgery compared to traditional surgery for autologous chondrocyte implantation (second generation). While in the second generation technique leads to form hyaline cartilage on the surface showing fibrosis and proliferation of small blood vessels (reactive fibrosis), by the use of periosteum, so that in this case it is advisable the use of membrane collagen

7. New proposals for repairing articular cartilage

In recent years they have sought new strategies for cartilage repair, with technological advances have currently been proposed the use of scaffolding or matrix on which cells can grow. Among the scaffolds used in the clinic (Table 2) are those that are based on collagen, hyaluronic acid and fibrin as these provide a substrate normally found in the structure of native articular cartilage. Collagen is a major extracellular matrix protein, exists to provide strength and stability to the connective tissues. At the clinic is used collagen I-III as scaffolds for growing chondrocytes in order to improve the structural and biological properties of the graft [116, 117] this is used as a sponge, foam, gel and membrane form, all these are subject to enzymatic degradation. Hyaluronic acid is another important component of articular cartilage matrix and is a glycosaminoglycan that is involved in homeostasis [118, 119] provides viscoelasticity to synovial fluid, is credited as a lubricant and shock absorbing properties, is essential for the correct structure of proteoglycans in articular cartilage. Between scaffolds containing hyaluronic acid is the Hylaff-11, which is an esterified derivative of hyaluronic acid and is used for growing chondrocytes in three dimensions, has been shown that when using this type of scaffold maintaining the chondrocyte phenotype, so that chondrocytes are capable of producing the proteins and molecules characteristic of a hyaline cartilage [120-122]. Fibrin is a protein involved in blood coagulation, is regarded as a biomaterial for cartilage repair, as can be found in gel form, having an adhesive function that is also biocompatible and biodegradable [123]. However in vivo studies in animals have shown to have low mechanical stability and can also trigger an immune response [124, 125], fibrin because this has only been used clinically to ensure healthy cartilage tissue-engineered the [126-128].

Based on the foregoing and which is being used in the clinic and according to results obtained in patients who have been treated with different biomaterials has been observed that although there is a suitable biomaterial that contributes to the production of extracellular matrix to provide the right conditions for chondrocyte cell differentiation. So it is necessary to propose new biomaterials that help produce extracellular matrix, capable of activating a cascade of signaling that can form a cartilage which has structural properties suitable for tissue repair, as well as having viscoelastic properties and to provide mechanical stability.

8. Cartilage tissue engineering and low scaffold successful

Many advances in the field of cartilage tissue engineering have been closely connected to the improved performance of biomaterials. Successful cartilage tissue engineering relies on four specific criteria: (1) cells, (2) signaling molecules, (3) biomaterials, and the (4) mechanical environment. Furthermore, they should be biocompatible, non-toxic, bioresorbable and highly permeable to facilitate mass transport [139].

The use of scaffolds to support replication of chondrocytes for production of cartilage in vitro has been the most common approach for tissue engineering of cartilage, however, despite the

Ref.	Biomaterial	Component	Method of autologous Chondrocyte transplantation	Results
[126, 129-132]	Carticel	Collagen I-III	2nd and 3rd generation	Three-dimensional multi-layer keeps the chondral phenotype
[113]	Matricel		2nd generation	
[133, 134]	CaReS®	Collagen I hydrogel	2nd generation	It presents a significant functional improvement as well as acting on the levels of pain.
[135-136]	Hyalograft-C		3rd generation	Maintaining the chondral phenotype, absence of inflammatory response, formation of hyaline cartilage
[137]	Hyalgan®	Hyaluronic acid	--------------	Indicated for the treatment of osteoarthritis of the knee, improves mobility and reduces pain.
[113]	Tisseel	Fibrin	3rd generation	Fibrin is an integral component of the extracellular matrix induced chondrocytes, so that the new cartilage is well integrated into the underlying subchondral bone. Moderate application of fibrin
[138]	Cartipatch	Alginate Hydrogel-agarose	--------	Hyaline cartilage was observed in eight of the 13 patients treated, clinical improvement at 2 years of treatment

Table 2. Biomaterials most used in the clinic, with different components for the repair of articular cartilage by autologous transplantation method of chondrocytes from second and third generation.

apparent simplicity of cartilage, to our knowledge, tissue engineered cartilage has not been successfully reached so far [140-142].

In theory, a scaffold for tissue engineering should have a three dimensional porous structure forming an interconnected porous network. These structures should be made of biocompatible and biodegradable materials capable to provide mechanical strength, support cells ingrowth, promote cells adhesion, uniform cell spreading, and conserve phenotypes and functional characteristics of transplanted cells [143,144]. Unfortunately, this list of requirements looks too long and hard to accomplish. Probably this is one of the main reasons of why the advances in cartilage engineering have been too slow. But also we should rethink these concepts in order to find shorter and easier pathways to find more efficient and effective tissue engineering methods.

The vast majority of scaffolds used in tissue engineering are solid sponge-like porous structures that are seeded with cells in a culture media. Analyzing this approach from the basic principles for the design of biomaterials, the biomimetism, easily we can find out that this process lacks of this basic concept. In natural tissues, cells grow in a physiological environment which is more like a gel medium than a porous scaffold, they do not form tissues by populating porous structures, but they do it by creating their own ECM starting from a gel-like environment. Following this line, many researchers are proposing the encapsulation of cells in hydrogels instead of using porous scaffolds, looking to improve the biomimetic environment for cells [145,146,147,148].

Besides biomimetism, sponge-like scaffolds provides only a two dimensional surface for cell attachment, although their structure is 3D, cells attach to the walls of the scaffold, thus changing completely the way they are integrated into natural tissues. On the other hand hydrogels are capable to provide a real 3D environment when cells are seeded (encapsulated) into them [149].

8.1. Hydrogels for articular cartilage tissue engineering

Hydrogels are water-swollen, cross-linked polymeric structures [150] that possess unique mechanical and chemical properties that make them very attractive for a variety of biomedical applications; actually there are no other materials capable to display characteristics too close to natural tissues such as Hydrogels. Therefore hydrogels have been considered as a key material in the development of new biomaterials for tissue engineering and artificial organs fabrication.

Their particular properties come from their structure, composed of swollen randomly cross-linked networks of rod-like polymer chains with water filling the interstitial spaces.[151] Water commonly comprises more than 80% of the total volume. The physical properties of hydrogels are determined by the polymer composition and concentration, the cross-linking density between polymer chains [152], polymerization conditions [153], the addition of hydrophobic monomers which may create regions of more dense coiled or entangled chains, the introduction of composite materials such as rubber or glass, the use of cross-linking agents such as glutaraldehyde, and the use of freeze-thawing procedures to induce partial crystallinity [154].

Hydrogels can be classified by the type of crosslinking: covalently or ionic cross-linked, physical gels, or entangled networks [155]. The two first are the most common gels. Physical gels are formed by non-covalent interactions, such as hydrogen bonding, and hydrophobic interactions [156]. Covalently or ionic cross linked gels are considerably more stable than physical gels and once they are formed they may not be re-melted again.

Hydrogels can be obtained from natural or synthetic polymers. Natural hydrogels come from proteins and polypeptides (commonly collagen and gelatin), polysaccharides (i.e. alginate, agarose, hyaluronic acid, fibrin, chitin and chitosan). On the other hand, synthetic polymers come from man-made materials such as polyester (i.e. poly L-lactic and polyglycolic acid, poly ε-caprolactone, polypropylene fumarate), polyethylene oxide, polyethylene glycol, polyvinyl alcohol, polyurethane, polydiol citrates, polyhydroxyethyl methacrylate, and many others polymers [157].

Although hydrogel scaffolding technologies plays a crucial role in cartilage tissue engineering, several studies has been shown low success cartilage tissue repair. They are unable to generate cartilaginous tissues with similar properties to native cartilage [141-142].

There are a number of reasons for scaffolds failure, we summarized some of them:

1. The scaffold architecture should be designed to mimic the depth-dependent heterogeneity of articular cartilage structure or to generate multiphasic scaffolds to promote the simultaneous growth of bone and cartilage with a stable interface for engineering osteochondral tissue.

2. However, manufacturing scaffolds technologies are limited and no optimum architectures have been produce yet.

3. The study of biological cartilage development is still growing.

4. Not enough knowledge about:

5. the role of chondrocyte ECM and their implications during chondrogenesis.

6. the role of adhesion molecules and signaling pathways during chondrogenesis.

7. Culture chondrocytes *in vitro* and density cells conditions in scaffolds.

8. Dynamic cartilage ECM and their Nanomechanical properties.

9. Chemical variables in cell-scaffolds interactions, among others.

8.2. Trends in hydrogel-scaffolding cartilage repair

However towards designing biomimetic native environments cartilage is still a challenge due articular cartilage is intricately organized and heterogeneous tissue. This tissue reveals a highly defined structural organization that can be subdivided into two domains, the cartilage zones and the organization of the extracellular matrix. In that sense the ECM of articular cartilage is a unique environment with complex heterogeneity and spatial conformation very difficult to mimic. One of the most notable variations in this tissue is the spatial organization of collagen network and cells arrangement. [141]. Moreover cartilage presents different morphology, gene expression, matrix spatial array between cultured populations isolated from distinct cartilage zones [142]. However, intensive researches have been focus on the development of an ideal scaffold material with versatile properties that actively contribute to cartilage repair [158]. In that regard, there have been several attempts trying to recreate the different zones in cartilage by different hydrogel fabrication technologies, giving as a result tridimensional homogeneous structures with little resemblance to the native organization in cartilage, so it is necessary to material scientists thinking in others design hydrogel-scaffolding strategies trying to biomimetic hierarchical structures capable to deliver bioactive molecules such as growth factors with an ideal mechanical response and mediated by adhesive molecules in order to have an integration tissue [159].

Currently strategies in the design of biomimetic cartilage hydrogels are governed by the use of collagen Type I and derived from porcine small intestine submucosa implants. Although the chondrocytes typically lose their phenotype, the gene expression patterns changed when they are removed from their native environment, so give them a proper environment is necessary to keep its phenotype of chondrocytes in different populations to recreate the zonal organization [160]. In addition, biological trials *in vitro* be made taking into account the cell density for each zone [161,162].

According with reference [163] concentrations of 12-25 million cells/cm^2 are needed to increase the matrix production and mechanical properties of human adult chondrocytes under static conditions. Nevertheless, material researches are focus on fabrication of three-dimensional artificial arrays in form of hydrogels using macromolecules present in the cartilage inter-territorial matrix and trying to mimic the distinct cartilage zonal [160]; however, no substantial data of the formation of cartilage are reported.

Others approaches in cartilage tissue engineering are the use of hydrogel culture employed mesenchymal stem cells (MSCs) and the use of bioreactors in order to provide the necessary biochemical and biomechanical stimulations to enhance chondrogenesis [164,165]. Due to the many mentioned limitations related to chondrocyte sources, there is much effort to explore better alternative cell sources. Desirable characteristics for such sources include accessibility, availability, and chondrogenic capacity. Consequently, stem cells such as adult mesenchymal stem cells (MSCs) have emerged as promising cell sources for articular cartilage tissue engineering. Chondrogenic potentials of MSCs from different tissues have also been investigated and compared. Specifically, MSCs from bone marrow are the most popular considering they are easily harvested (via the iliac crest) and have good chondrogenic potential. Many in vitro and in vivo studies have revealed promising results of marrowderived MSCs combined with various biomaterials or growth factors for repairing cartilage defects [164,166]. Recently, Johnson et al. describe the discovery and characterization of kartogenin, a small molecule that induced stem cells to take on the characteristics of chondrocytes and improves joint function and promotes the regeneration of cartilage in vivo in two rodent models of chronic and acute joint [166].

Mechanical stresses are an important factor of chondrocyte function as they stimulate them to increase the synthesis of ECM components. In cartilage culturing processes the main types of mechanical forces currently being investigated are hydrostatic pressure, direct compression, shear environments [167, 168].

Finally, to better recapitulate the ECM environment for cartilage tissue engineering, research-ers have to introduce several biological signals, including chondroitin sulfate (CS), hyaluronic acid (HA), and collagen type I and II, into tissue-engineered scaffolds to encourage tissue specificity [169]. CS, hyaluronic acid, and collagen type II have been shown to promote or enhance chondrogenesis of mesenchymal stem cells (MSCs) in hydrogel-based culture systems. In addition to the physical cues of native matrix, cells are exposed to an array of biological cues throughout the ECM that direct cellular behavior.

Cells are constantly interacting with the surrounding ECM, which gives rise to a dynamic transfer of information between the extracellular and intracellular space. In addition, biological trials *in vitro* be made taking into account the cell density for each zone [169].

Tissue engineering should be the best way to achieve successful cartilage regeneration by combining novel biologically inspired scaffolds approaches, nanotechnology, cell sources such as stem cells, chondrogenic factors, and physical stimuli [165].

Author details

Zaira Y. García-Carvajal[1], David Garciadiego-Cázares[1], Carmen Parra-Cid[1], Rocío Aguilar-Gaytán[1], Cristina Velasquillo [3], Clemente Ibarra[1,2] and Javier S. Castro Carmona[4]

1 Tissue Engineering, Cell Therapy and Regenerative Medicine Unit. Instituto Nacional de Rehabilitación, Secretaria de Salud. Mexico city, Mexico

2 Orthopaedic Surgery and Arthroscopy Servicie, Instituto Nacional de Rehabilitación, Secretaria de Salud. Mexico city, Mexico

3 Biotechnology Laboratory. Centro Nacional de Investigación y Atención al Quemado. Instituto Nacional de Rehabilitación, Secretaria de Salud. Mexico city, Mexico

4 Instituto de Ingenieria y Tecnologia. Universidad Autónoma de Ciudad Juárez, Juarez City, Chihuahua, Mexico

References

[1] Buckwalter, J.A., J.A. Martin, and T.D. Brown, Perspectives on chondrocyte mechanobiology and osteoarthritis. Biorheology 2004; 41(3-4):593-6.

[2] Benedek, T.G., A history of the understanding of cartilage. Osteoarthritis Cartilage 2006; 14(3) 203-9.

[3] Hunziker, E.B., T.M. Quinn, and H.J. Hauselmann, Quantitative structural organization of normal adult human articular cartilage. Osteoarthritis Cartilage, 2002; 10(7): 564-72, 2002.

[4] Goldring, M.B., Update on the biology of the chondrocyte and new approaches to treating cartilage diseases. Best Pract Res Clin Rheumatol, 2006; 20(5):1003-25.

[5] Goldring, M.B. and S.R. Goldring, Osteoarthritis. J Cell Physiol, 213(3): p. 626-34, 2007.

[6]   Saxne, T., et al., Inflammation is a feature of the disease process in early knee joint osteoarthritis. Rheumatology (Oxford), 2003; 42(7): 903-4.

[7]   Sridhar, M.S., et al., Obesity and symptomatic osteoarthritis of the knee. J Bone Joint Surg Br, 94(4): p. 433-40, 2012.

[8]   Issa, R.I. and T.M. Griffin. Pathobiology of obesity and osteoarthritis: integrating biomechanics and inflammation. Pathobiol Aging Age Relat Dis. 2012; 9 (2):17470.

[9]   Ewers, B.J., et al., The extent of matrix damage and chondrocyte death in mechanically traumatized articular cartilage explants depend on rate of loading. J Orthop Res, 2001;19(5): 779-84.

[10] Tetsworth, K. and D. Paley, Malalignment and degenerative arthropathy. Orthop Clin North Am, 1994; 25(3): 367-77.

[11] Cerejo, R., et al., The influence of alignment on risk of knee osteoarthritis progression according to baseline stage of disease. Arthritis Rheum, 2002; 46(10):2632-6

[12] Tanamas, S., et al., Does knee malalignment increase the risk of development and progression of knee osteoarthritis? A systematic review. Arthritis Rheum, 2009; 61(4): 459-67.

[13] Fukuda, Y., et al., Impact load transmission of the knee joint-influence of leg alignment and the role of meniscus and articular cartilage. Clin Biomech (Bristol, Avon), 2000; 15(7):516-21.

[14] Lanzer, W.L. and G. Komenda, Changes in articular cartilage after meniscectomy. Clin Orthop Relat Res, 1990;252: 41-8.

[15] Musahl, V., et al., The effect of medial versus lateral meniscectomy on the stability of the anterior cruciate ligament-deficient knee. Am J Sports Med, 2010;38(8):1591-7.

[16] Berthiaume, M.J., et al., Meniscal tear and extrusion are strongly associated with progression of symptomatic knee osteoarthritis as assessed by quantitative magnetic resonance imaging. Ann Rheum Dis, 2005; 64(4): 556-63.

[17] Buckwalter, J.A., Articular cartilage injuries. Clin Orthop Relat Res, 2002; 402:21-37.

[18] Heir, S., et al., Focal cartilage defects in the knee impairs quality of life as much as severe osteoarthritis: a comparison of knee injury and osteoarthritis outcome score in 4 patient categories scheduled for knee surgery. Am J Sports Med, 2010; 38(2): 231-7.

[19] Lohmander, L.S., et al., The long-term consequence of anterior cruciate ligament and meniscus injuries: osteoarthritis. Am J Sports Med, 2007; 35(10):1756-69.

[20] Versier, G. and F. Dubrana, Treatment of knee cartilage defect in 2010. Orthop Traumatol Surg Res, 2011; 97(8 Suppl): S140-53.

[21] Eyre, D., Collagen of articular cartilage. Arthritis Res, 2002. 4(1): 30-5.

[22] Hyc, A., et al., The morphology and selected biological properties of articular cartilage. Ortop Traumatol Rehabil, 2001; 3(2): 151-62.

[23] Poole, A.R., et al., Composition and structure of articular cartilage: a template for tissue repair. Clin Orthop Relat Res, 2001; 391 Suppl: S26-33.

[24] Korhonen, R.K., et al., Importance of collagen orientation and depth-dependent fixed
charge densities of cartilage on mechanical behavior of chondrocytes. J Biomech Eng,
2008; 130(2): 021003.

[25] Huber, M., S. Trattnig, and F. Lintner, Anatomy, biochemistry, and physiology of articular cartilage. Invest Radiol, 2000; 35(10): 573-80.

[26] Schrobback, K., et al., Effects of oxygen on zonal marker expression in human articular chondrocytes. Tissue Eng Part A, 2012; 18(9-10): 920-33.

[27] Mobasheri, A., et al., Hypoxia inducible factor-1 and facilitative glucose transporters
GLUT1 and GLUT3: putative molecular components of the oxygen and glucose sensing apparatus in articular chondrocytes. Histol Histopathol, 2005; 20(4):1327-38.

[28] Martel-Pelletier, J., et al., Cartilage in normal and osteoarthritis conditions. Best Pract
Res Clin Rheumatol, 2008; 22(2): 351-84.

[29] Heijink, A., et al., Biomechanical considerations in the pathogenesis of osteoarthritis
of the knee. Knee Surg Sports Traumatol Arthrosc, 2012; 20(3): 423-35.

[30] Silver, F.H., G. Bradica, and A. Tria, Relationship among biomechanical, biochemical,
and cellular changes associated with osteoarthritis. Crit Rev Biomed Eng, 2001; 29(4):
373-91.

[31] Guilak, F., et al., The pericellular matrix as a transducer of biomechanical and biochemical signals in articular cartilage. Ann N Y Acad Sci, 2006;1068:498-512.

[32] Guilak, F., et al., The deformation behavior and mechanical properties of chondrocytes in articular cartilage. Osteoarthritis Cartilage, 1999; 7(1): 59-70.

[33] Eyre, D.R., M.A. Weis, and J.J. Wu, Articular cartilage collagen: an irreplaceable
framework? Eur Cell Mater, 2006; 12: 57-63.

[34] Heinegard, D., Proteoglycans and more--from molecules to biology. Int J Exp Pathol,
2009; 90(6): 575-86.

[35] Gentili, C. and R. Cancedda, Cartilage and bone extracellular matrix. Curr Pharm
Des, 2009; 15(12): 1334-48.

[36] Kim, S.H., J. Turnbull, and S. Guimond, Extracellular matrix and cell signalling: the
dynamic cooperation of integrin, proteoglycan and growth factor receptor. J Endocri-
nol, 2011; 209(2):139-51.

[37] Shakibaei, M., C. Csaki, and A. Mobasheri, Diverse roles of integrin receptors in articular cartilage. Adv Anat Embryol Cell Biol, 2008; 197:1-60.

[38] Vonwil, D., et al., An RGD-restricted substrate interface is sufficient for the adhesion, growth and cartilage forming capacity of human chondrocytes. Eur Cell Mater, 2010; 20: 316-28.

[39] Redini, F., Structure and regulation of articular cartilage proteoglycan expression. Pathol Biol, 2001; 49(4): 364-75.

[40] Bertrand, J., et al., Molecular mechanisms of cartilage remodelling in osteoarthritis. Int J Biochem Cell Biol, 2010; 42(10):1594-601.

[41] Struglics, A., et al., Human osteoarthritis synovial fluid and joint cartilage contain both aggrecanase- and matrix metalloproteinase-generated aggrecan fragments. Osteoarthritis Cartilage, 2006; 14(2): 101-13.

[42] Olsen, B. R. Morphogenesis: collagen it takes and bone it makes. Curr Biol 1996; 6, 645–647.

[43] Kannu, P., Bateman, J. F., Belluoccio, D., Fosang, A. J. & Savarirayan, R. Employing molecular genetics of chondrodysplasias to inform the study of osteoarthritis. Arthritis Rheum 2009; 60, 325–334.

[44] Barsh, G. S. & Byers, P. H. Reduced secretion of structurally abnormal type I procollagen in a form of osteogenesis imperfecta. PNAS USA 1981; 78, 5142–5146.

[45] Chan, D. & Jacenko, O. Phenotypic and biochemical consequences of collagen X mutations in mice and humans. Matrix Biol 1998; 17, 169–184.

[46] Chen, F. H., Thomas, A. O., Hecht, J. T., Goldring, M. B. & Lawler, J. Cartilage oligomeric matrix protein/thrombospondin 5 supports chondrocyte attachment through interaction with integrins. J Biol Chem 2005; 280, 32655–32661.

[47] Storm, E. E. et al. Limb alterations in brachypodism mice due to mutations in a new member of the TGF beta-superfamily. Nature 1994; 368, 639–643.

[48] Gualeni, B. et al. Defective proteoglycan sulfation of the growth plate zones causes reduced chondrocyte proliferation via an altered Indian hedgehog signalling. Matrix Biol 2020; 29, 453–460.

[49] Hargus, G. et al. Loss of Sox9 function results in defective chondrocyte differentiation of mouse embryonic stem cells in vitro. Int J Dev Biol 2008; 52, 323–332.

[50] Zhao, Q., Eberspaecher, H., Lefebvre, V. & de Crombrugghe, B. Parallel expression of Sox9 and Col2a1 in cells undergoing chondrogenesis. Dev Dyn 1997; 209, 377–386.

[51] Lefebvre, V. & Smits, P. Transcriptional control of chondrocyte fate and differentiation. Birth Defect Res C 2005; 75, 200–212.

[52] Vu, T. H. & Werb, Z. Matrix metalloproteinases: effectors of development and normal physiology. Genes Dev 2000; 14, 2123–2133.

[53] Chuang, C. Y. et al. The cartilage matrix molecule components produced by human foetal cartilage rudiment cells within scaffolds and the role of exogenous growth factors. Biomaterials 2012; 33, 4078–4088.

[54] Hynes, R. O. The extracellular matrix: not just pretty fibrils. Science 2009; 326, 1216–1219.

[55] Hirsch, M. S., Lunsford, L. E., Trinkaus-Randall, V. & Svoboda, K. K. Chondrocyte survival and differentiation in situ are integrin mediated. Dev Dyn 1997; 210, 249–263.

[56] Shakibaei, M. & Merker, H. J. Beta1-integrins in the cartilage matrix. Cell Tissue Res 1999; 296, 565–573.

[57] Bonnet, C. S. & Walsh, D. A. Osteoarthritis, angiogenesis and inflammation. Rheumatology 20005; 44, 7–16.

[58] Jubeck, B., Muth, E., Gohr, C. M. & Rosenthal, A. K. Type II collagen levels correlate with mineralization by articular cartilage vesicles. Arthritis Rheum 2009; 60, 2741–2746.

[59] Little, C. B. et al. Matrix metalloproteinase 13-deficient mice are resistant to osteoarthritic cartilage erosion but not chondrocyte hypertrophy or osteophyte development. Arthritis Rheum 2009; 60, 3723–3733.

[60] Majumdar, M. K. et al. Double-knockout of ADAMTS-4 and ADAMTS-5 in mice results in physiologically normal animals and prevents the progression of osteoarthritis. Arthritis Rheum 2007; 56, 3670–3674.

[61] Xu, L. et al. Increased expression of the collagen receptor discoidin domain receptor 2 in articular cartilage as a key event in the pathogenesis of osteoarthritis. Arthritis Rheum 2007; 56, 2663–2673.

[62] van der Kraan, P. M., Blaney Davidson, E. N., Blom, A. & van den Berg, W. B. TGF-beta signaling in chondrocyte terminal differentiation and osteoarthritis: modulation and integration of signaling pathways through receptor-Smads. Osteoarthritis and Cartilage 2009; 17, 1539–1545.

[63] Yang, X. et al. TGF-{beta}/Smad3 signals repress chondrocyte hypertrophic differentiation and are required for maintaining articular cartilage. J Cell Biol 2001; 153, 35.

[64] Diarra, D. et al. Dickkopf-1 is a master regulator of joint remodeling. Nat Med 2007; 13, 156–163.

[65] Luyten, F. P., Tylzanowski, P. & Lories, R. J. Wnt signaling and osteoarthritis. Bone 2009; 44, 522–527.

[66] Mateescu, R. G., Todhunter, R. J., Lust, G. & Burton-Wurster, N. Increased MIG-6 mRNA transcripts in osteoarthritic cartilage. Biochem Biophys Res Commun 2005; 332, 482–486.

[67] McGlashan, S. R., Haycraft, C. J., Jensen, C. G., Yoder, B. K. & Poole, C. A. Articular cartilage and growth plate defects are associated with chondrocyte cytoskeletal abnormalities in Tg737orpk mice lacking the primary cilia protein polaris. Matrix Biol 2007; 26, 234–246.

[68] Poole, A. R. et al. Type II collagen degradation and its regulation in articular cartilage in osteoarthritis. Ann Rheum Dis 2002; 61 Suppl 2, ii78–81.

[69] Ionescu, A. M. et al. PTHrP modulates chondrocyte differentiation through AP-1 and CREB signaling. J Biol Chem 2001; 276, 11639–11647.

[70] Ohbayashi, N. et al. FGF18 is required for normal cell proliferation and differentiation during osteogenesis and chondrogenesis. Genes Dev 2002; 16, 870–879.

[71] Lanske, B. et al. PTH/PTHrP receptor in early development and Indian hedgehog-regulated bone growth. Science 1996; 273, 663–666.

[72] Jay, G. D., Torres, J. R., Warman, M. L., Laderer, M. C. & Breuer, K. S. The role of lubricin in the mechanical behavior of synovial fluid. PNAS USA 2007; 104, 6194–6199.

[73] Dowthwaite, G. P., Edwards, J. C. & Pitsillides, A. A. An essential role for the interaction between hyaluronan and hyaluronan binding proteins during joint development. J Histochem Cytochem 1998; 46, 641–651.

[74] Koyama, E. et al. Synovial joint formation during mouse limb skeletogenesis: roles of Indian hedgehog signaling. Ann N Y Acad Sci 2007; 1116, 100–112.

[75] Archer, C. W., Dowthwaite, G. P. & Francis-West, P. H. Development of synovial joints. Birth Defect Res C 2003; 69, 144–155.

[76] Hartmann, C. & Tabin, C. J. Wnt-14 plays a pivotal role in inducing synovial joint formation in the developing appendicular skeleton. Cell 2001; 104, 341–351.

[77] Brunet, L. J., McMahon, J. A., McMahon, A. P. & Harland, R. M. Noggin, cartilage morphogenesis, and joint formation in the mammalian skeleton. Science 1998; 280, 1455–1457.

[78] Garciadiego-Cázares, D., Rosales, C., Katoh, M. & Chimal-Monroy, J. Coordination of chondrocyte differentiation and joint formation by alpha5beta1 integrin in the developing appendicular skeleton. Development 2004; 131, 4735–4742.

[79] Jones, D. C. et al. Uncoupling of growth plate maturation and bone formation in mice lacking both Schnurri-2 and Schnurri-3. PNAS USA 2010; 107, 8254–8258.

[80] Wu, Q., Zhang, Y. & Chen, Q. Indian hedgehog is an essential component of mechanotransduction complex to stimulate chondrocyte proliferation. J Biol Chem 2001; 276, 35290–35296.

[81] Kamekura, S. et al. Contribution of runt-related transcription factor 2 to the pathogenesis of osteoarthritis in mice after induction of knee joint instability. Arthritis Rheum 2006; 54, 2462–2470.

[82] Ornitz, D. M. & Marie, P. J. FGF signaling pathways in endochondral and intramembranous bone development and human genetic disease. Genes Dev 2002; 16, 1446–1465.

[83] Legeai-Mallet, L., Benoist-Lasselin, C., Delezoide, A. L., Munnich, A. & Bonaventure, J. Fibroblast growth factor receptor 3 mutations promote apoptosis but do not alter chondrocyte proliferation in thanatophoric dysplasia. J Biol Chem 1998; 273, 13007–13014.

[84] Francis-West, P. H., Parish, J., Lee, K. & Archer, C. W. BMP/GDF-signalling interactions during synovial joint development. Cell Tissue Res 1999; 296, 111–119.

[85] Francis-West, P. H. et al. Mechanisms of GDF-5 action during skeletal development. Development 1999; 126, 1305–1315.

[86] Reddi, A. H. Cartilage morphogenetic proteins: role in joint development, homoeostasis, and regeneration. Ann Rheum Dis 2003; 62 Suppl 2, ii73–8.

[87] Dell'Accio, F. et al. Activation of WNT and BMP signaling in adult human articular cartilage following mechanical injury. Arthritis Res Ther 2006; 8, R139.

[88] Dowthwaite, G. P. et al. The surface of articular cartilage contains a progenitor cell population. J Cell Sci 2004; 117, 889–897.

[89] Buckwalter J. A and Mankin H. J. "Articular cartilage: tissuedesign and chondrocyte-matrix interactions," Instructional course lectures, 1998 vol. 47, pp. 477–486.

[90] Hunziker EB. Articular cartilage repair: basic science and clinical progress. A review of the current status and prospects. Osteoarthritis Cartilage. 2002 Jun; 10(6):432-63.

[91] Noyes FR, Bassett RW, Grood ES, Butler DL. Arthroscopy in acute traumatic hemarthrosis of the knee. Incidence of anterior cruciate tears and other injuries. J Bone Joint Surg Am. 1980 Jul;62 (5):687-95, 757.

[92] Hjelle K, Solheim E, Strand T, Muri R, Brittberg M. Articular cartilage defects in 1,000 kneearthroscopies. Arthroscopy, 2002 18:730-734.

[93] Curl WW, Krome J, Gordon ES, Rushing J, Smith BP, Poehling GG.Cartilage injuries: a review of 31,516 knee arthroscopies. Arthroscopy, 1997 13:456-460.

[94] Pridie K. A method of resurfacing osteoarthritis knee joints. J bone joint surg. br. 1959 41:618-619.

[95] Steadman JR, Rodkey WG, Briggs KK, Rodrigo JJ. The microfracture technician the management of complete cartilage defects in the knee joint. Orthopedic. 1999 28:26-32.

[96]   Magnuson PB. The classic: Joint debridement: surgical treatment of degenerative ar-
       thritis. Clin Orthop Relat Res. 1974 Jun; (101):4-12.

[97]   Pridie K. A method of resurfacing osteoarthritis knee joints. J bone joint surg. br. 1959
       41:618-619.

[98]   Trattnig S, Pinker K, Krestan C, Plank C, Millington S, Marlovits S. Matrix-based au-
       tologous chondrocyte implantation for cartilage repair with HyalograftC: two-year
       follow-up by magnetic resonance imaging. Eur J Radiol. 2006 Jan;57(1):9-15.

[99]   Knutsen G, Drogset JO, Engebretsen L, Grøntvedt T, Isaksen V, Ludvigsen TC, Rob-
       erts S, Solheim E, Strand T, Johansen O. A. Randomized trial comparing autologous
       chondrocyte implantation with microfracture. Findings at five years. J Bone Joint
       Surg Am 2007 Oct; 89(10):2105-12.

[100] Lassandro F, Romano S, Ragozzino A, Rossi G, Valente T, Ferrara I, Romano L,
       Grassi R. Role of helical CT in diagnosis of gallstone ileus and related conditions.
       AJR Am J Roentgenol. 2005 Nov. 185 (5):1159-65,

[101] Knutsen G, Engebretsen L, Ludvigsen TC, Drogset JO, Grøntvedt T, Solheim E,
       Strand T, Roberts S, Isaksen V, Johansen O. 2004. Autologous chondrocyte implanta-
       tion compared with microfracture in the knee. A randomized trial. J Bone Joint Surg
       Am. 2004 Mar; 86-A(3):455-64.

[102] Henderson I, Lavigne P, Valenzuela H, Oakes B. Autologous chondrocyte implanta-
       tion: superior biologic properties of hyaline cartilage repairs. Clin Orthop Relat Res.
       2007 Feb; 455:253-61, 2007.

[103] Hallal PC, Wells JC, Bertoldi AD, Gazalle FK, Silva MC, Domingues MR, Carret ML,
       Araújo CL, Gigante DP. A shift in the epidemiology of low body mass index in Bra-
       zilian adults. Eur J Clin Nutr. 2005 Sep; 59 (9):1002-6.

[104] Knutsen G, Drogset JO, Engebretsen L, Grøntvedt T, Isaksen V, Ludvigsen TC, Rob-
       erts S, Solheim E, Strand T, Johansen O. A. Randomized trial comparing autologous
       chondrocyte implantation with microfracture. Findings at five years. J Bone Joint
       Surg Am. 2007 Oct; 89 (10):2105-12.

[105] Leumann A, Wiewiorski M, Egelhof T, Rasch H, Magerkurth O, Candrian C, Schae-
       fer DJ, Martin I, Jakob M, Valderrabano V. Radiographic evaluation of frontal talar
       edge configuration for osteochondral plug transplantation. Clin Anat. 2009 Mar;
       22(2):261-6.

[106] Reguzzoni M, Manelli A, Ronga M, Raspanti M, Grassi FA. Histology and ultrastruc-
       ture of a tissue-engineered collagen meniscus before and after implantation. J Bi-
       omed Mater Res B Appl. Biomater. 2005 Aug ;74 (2):808-16.

[107] Hangody L, Kish G, Kárpáti Z, Szerb I, Udvarhelyi I. Arthroscopic autogenousosteo-
       chondralmosaicplasty for the treatment of femoral condylar articular defects. A pre-
       liminary report. Knee Surg Sports Traumatol Arthrosc. 1997;5 (4):262-7.

[108] Coen G, Moscaritolo E, Catalano C, Lavini R, Nofroni I, Ronga G, Sardella D, Zacca-
ria A, Cianci R. Atherosclerotic renal artery stenosis: one year outcome of total and
separate kidney function following stenting. BMC Nephrol. 2004 Oct 15;5:15.

[109] Richardson JB, Caterson B, Evans EH, Ashton BA, Roberts S. 1999. Repair of human
articular cartilage after implantation of autologous chondrocytes. J Bone Joint Surg
Br. 1999 Nov;81(6):1064-8.

[110] Brittberg M, Lindahl A, Nilsson A, Ohlsson C, Isaksson O, Peterson L. Treatment of
deep cartilage defects in the knee with autologous chondrocyte transplantation. N
Engl J Med. 1994 Oct 6; 331(14):889-95.

[111] Franceschi F, Longo UG, Ruzzini L, Marinozzi A, Maffulli N, Denaro V. Simultaneous arthroscopic implantation of autologous chondrocytes and high tibial osteotomy
for tibialchondral defects in the varus knee. Knee. 2008 Aug;15 (4):309-13.

[112] Bahuaud J, Maitrot RC, Bouvet R, Kerdiles N, Tovagliaro F, Synave J, Buisson P,
Thierry JF, Versier A, Romanet JP, Chauvin F, Gillet JP, Allizard JP, de Belenet H. Implantation of autologous chondrocytes for cartilagenous lesions in young patients. A
study of 24 cases. Chirurgie. 1998 Dec;123 (6):568-71.

[113] Bartlett W, Skinner JA, Gooding CR, Carrington RW, Flanagan AM, Briggs TW, Bentley G. Autologous chondrocyte implantation versus matrix-induced autologous
chondrocyte implantation for osteochondral defects of the knee: a prospective, randomised study. J Bone Joint Surg Br. 2005 May;87 (5):640-5.

[114] Barlic A, Drobnic M, Malicev E, Kregar-Velikonja N. Quantitative analysis of gene
expression in human articular chondrocytes assigned for autologous implantation. J
Orthop Res. 2008 Jun;26(6):847-53.

[115] Masri M, Lombardero G, Velasquillo C, Martínez V, Neri R, Villegas H, Ibarra C. Ma-
trix-encapsulation cell-seeding technique to prevent cell detachment during arthroscopic implantation of matrix-induced autologous chondrocytes. Arthroscopy.
2007Aug; 23(8):877-83.

[116] Chaipinyo K, Oakes BW, Van Damme MP. The use of debrided human articular cartilage for autologous chondrocyte implantation: maintenance of chondrocyte differentiation andproliferation in type I collagen gels. J Orthop Res. 2004 22:446–455.

[117] Grande DA, Halberstadt C, Naughton G, Schwartz R, Manji R. Evaluation of matrix
scaffolds for tissue engineering of articular cartilage grafts. J Biomed Mater Res. 1997
34:211–220.

[118] Chen WY, Abatangelo G. Functions of hyaluronan in wound repair. Wound Repair
Regen. 19997:79–89.

[119] Marcacci M, Berruto M, Brocchetta D, Delcogliano A, Ghinelli D, Gobbi A, Kon E,
Pederzini L, Rosa D, Sacchetti GL, Stefani G, Zanasi S. Articular cartilage engineering
with Hyalograft C: 3-year clinical results. Clin Orthop Relat Res.2005 435:96–105.

[120]   Aigner J, Tegeler J, Hutzler P, Campoccia D, Pavesio A, Hammer C, Kastenbauer E, Naumann A. Cartilage tissue engineering with novel nonwoven structured biomaterial based on hyaluronic acid benzyl ester. J Biomed Mater Res. 1998 42:172–181.

[121]   Brun P, Abatangelo G, Radice M, Zacchi V, Guidolin D, Daga Gordini D, Cortivo R. Chondrocyte aggregation and reorganization into three-dimensional scaffolds. J Biomed Mater Res. 1999 46:337–346.

[122]   Grigolo B, Lisignoli G, Piacentini A, FioriniM, Gobbi P,Mazzotti G, Duca M, Pavesio A, Facchini A. Evidence for redifferentiation of human chondrocytes grown on a hyaluronan-based biomaterial (HYAff 11): molecular, immunohistochemical and ultrastructural analysis. Biomaterials. 2002 23:1187–1195.

[123]   Kirilak Y, Pavlos NJ, Willers CR, Han R, Feng H, Xu J, Asokananthan N, Stewart GA, Henry P, Wood D, Zheng MH. Fibrin sealant promotes migration and proliferation of human articular chondrocytes: possible involvement of thrombin and protease-activated receptors. Int J Mol Med. 2006 17:551–558.

[124]   Van Susante JL, Buma P, Schuman L, Homminga GN, van den Berg WB, Veth RP. Resurfacing potential of heterologous chondrocytes suspended in fibrin glue in large full-thickness defects of femoral articular cartilage: an experimental study in the goat. Biomaterials. 1999 20:1167–1175.

[125]   Kawabe N, Yoshinao M. The repair of full-thickness articular cartilage defects. Immune responses to reparative tissue formed by llogeneic growth plate chondrocyte implants. Clin Orthop Relat Res. 1991 268:279–293.

[126]   Cherubino P, Grassi FA, Bulgheroni P, Ronga M. Autologous chondrocyte implantation using a bilayer collagen membrane: a preliminary report. J Orthop. Surg. 2003 11:10–15.

[127]   Pavesio A, Abatangelo G, Borrione A, Brocchetta D, Hollander AP, Kon E, Torasso F, Zanasi S, Marcacci M. Hyaluronan- based scaffolds (Hyalograft C) in the treatment of knee cartilage defects: preliminary clinical findings. Novartis Found Symp. 2003 249:203–217.

[128]   Visna P, Pasa L, Cizma´r I, Hart R, Hoch J. Treatment of deep cartilage defects of the knee using autologous chondrograft transplantation and by abrasive techniques–a randomized controlled study. Acta Chir Belg. 2004 104:709–714.

[129]   Gikas PD, Bayliss L, Bentley G, Briggs TW. An overview of autologous chondrocyte implantation .J Bone Joint Surg. Br. 2009 Aug; 91(8):997-1006.

[130]   Manfredini M, Zerbinati F, Gildone A, Faccini R. Autologous chondrocyte implantation: a comparison between an open periosteal-covered and an arthroscopic matrix-guided technique. Acta Orthop. Belg. 2007 73:207–218.

[131] Behrens P, Bitter T, Kurz B, Russlies M. Matrix-associated autologous chondrocyte transplantation/implantation (MACT/MACI)-5-year follow-up. Knee. 2006 13:194–202.

[132] Bartlett W, Gooding CR, Carrington RW, Skinner JA, Briggs TW, Bentley G. Autologous chondrocyte implantation at the knee using a bilayer collagen membrane with bone graft. A preliminary report. J Bone Joint Surg. Br. 2005 Mar; 87(3):330-2.

[133] Schneider U, Rackwitz L, Andereya S, Siebenlist S, Fensky F, Reichert J, Löer I, Barthel T, Rudert M, Nöth U. A prospective multicenter study on the outcome of type I collagen hydrogel-based autologous chondrocyte implantation (CaReS) for the repair of articular cartilage defects in the knee. Am J Sports Med. 2011 Dec; 39 (12):2558-65.

[134] Rackwitz L, Schneider U, Andereya S, Siebenlist S, Reichert JC, Fensky F, Arnhold J, Löer I, Grossstück R, Zinser W, Barthel T, Rudert M, Nth U. Reconstruction of osteochondral defects with a collagen I hydrogel. Results of a prospective multicenter study. Orthopade. 2012 Apr; 41(4):268-79.

[135] Della Villa S, Kon E, Filardo G, Ricci M, Vincentelli F, Delcogliano M, Marcacci M. Does intensive rehabilitation permit early return to sport without compromising the clinical outcome after arthroscopic autologous chondrocyte implantation in highly competitive athletes? Am J Sports Med. 2010 Jan; 38(1):68-77.

[136] Grigolo B, Lisignoli G, Piacentini A, FioriniM, Gobbi P,Mazzotti G, Duca M, Pavesio A, Facchini A. Evidence for redifferentiation of human chondrocytes grown on a hyaluronan-based biomaterial (HYAff 11): molecular, immunohistochemical and ultrastructural analysis. Biomaterials. 2002 23:1187–1195.

[137] Solchaga LA, Dennis JE, Goldberg VM, Caplan .I. Hyaluronic acid-based polymers as cell carriers for tissue engineered repair of bone and cartilage.J Orthop. Res. 1999 Mar; 17(2):205-13.

[138] Selmi TA, Verdonk P, Chambat P, Dubrana F, Potel JF, Barnouin L, Neyret P. Autologous chondrocyte implantation in a novel alginate-agarose hydrogel: outcome at two years. J Bone Joint Surg. Br. 2008 90:597-604.

[139] Kyoung-Hwan Choi, Byung Hyune Choi, So Ra Park, Byoung Ju Kim, Byoung-Hyun Min. The chondrogenic differentiation of mesenchymal stem cells on an extracellular matrix scaffold derived from porcine chondrocytes. Biomaterials 2010; 31: 5355-5365.

[140] Nicodemus GD, Bryant SJ. Cell Encapsulation in Biodegradable Hydrogels for Tissue Engineering Applications. Tissue Eng Part B Rev. 2008;14 (2): 149-65.

[141] Ge Z, Li C, Heng BC, Cao G, Yang Z. Functional biomaterials for cartilage regeneration. J Biomed Mater Res A. 2012; 100 (9):2526-36.

[142] Coates Emily E, Fisher John P. Robert L. In Burdick, Jason A.; Mauck, editors. Biomaterials for Tissue Engineering Applications: A Review of the Past and Future Trends-

Cartilage Engineering: Current Status and Future Trends, Springer;2011; 279-306. http://rd.springer.com/book/10.1007/978-3-7091-0385-2/page/1

[143] Chung-Hwan B, Ye-Jeung K. Characteristics of Tissue-Engineered Cartilage on Macroporous Biodegradable PLGA Scaffold. Laryngoscope. 2006 116: 1829–1834.

[144] [2]Diaz-Romero J, Gaillard JP, Grogan SP, Nesic D, Trub T, Mainil-Varlet P. Immunophenotypic analysis of human articular chondrocytes: Changes in surface markers associated with cell expansion in monolayer culture. J Cell Physiol. 2005 202:731–742.

[145] Hiroyuki Miyajima et al. Hydrogel-based biomimetic enviroment for in vitro modulation of branching morphogenesis. Biomaterials. 2011 32: 6754-6763.

[146] Sun-Young C, Cross D, and Wang C. Facile Synthesis and Characterization of Disulfide-Cross-Linked Hyaluronic Acid Hydrogels for Protein Delivery and Cell Encapsulation. Biomacromolecules. 2011 12: 1126–1136.

[147] Leda Clouda, et al. Thermoresponsive, in situ cross-linkable hydrogels based on N-isopropylacrylamide: Fabrication, characterization and mesenchymal stem cell encapsulation. Acta biomateriala. 2011 7: 1460-1467.

[148] Vinatier C, Guicheuxa J, Daculsi G, Layrolle P, and Weiss P. Cartilage and bone tissue engineering using Hydrogels. Bio-Medical Materials and Engineering. 2006 16.

[149] Nicola C. Hunt and Liam M. Grover. Cell encapsulation using biopolymer gels for regenerative Medicine. Biotechnol Lett. 2010 32:733–742.

[150] Peppas, N.A. Hydrogels in medicine and pharmacy. 1987 CRC Press, Boca Raton, FL.

[151] Sandra Cram, Hugh Brown, Geoff Spinks, Dominique Hourdet, Costantino Creton. Hydrophobically Modified Acrylamide Based Hydrogels Proc. of SPIE. 2005 5648:153-162.

[152] Kong HJ, Kim CJ, Huebsch N, Weitz D, and Mooney DJ. Noninvasive Probing of the Spatial Organization of Polymer Chains in Hydrogels Using Fluorescence Resonance Energy Transfer (FRET) J. AM. CHEM. SOC. 2007 129(15): 4518.

[153] Stammen JA, Williams S, Ku DN, Guldberg RE. Mechanical properties of a novel PVA hydrogel in shear and unconfined compression. Biomaterials. 2001 22:799-806.

[154] Zheng-Qiu G, Jiu-Mei X, Xiang-Hong Z. The development of artificial articular cartilage - PVA-hydrogel. Biomed Mater Engng. 1998 8:75-81.

[155] Kavanagh GM & Ross-Murphy SB. Rheological characterisation of polymer gels. Progress in Polymer Science. 1998 23:533-562.

[156] Barrangou LM, Daubert CR, Foegeding EA. Textural properties of agarose gels. I. Rheological and fracture properties. Food Hydrocolloids. 2006 20:184-195.

[157] Peppas NA. Hydrogels. In: Ratner B. (ed.) Biomaterial Science. An introduction to materials in medicine. Elsevier Academic Press. San Diego, Cal. 2004 p.100-112.

[158] Klein TJ, Malda J, Sah RL, Hutmacher DW. Tissue Engineering of Articular Cartilage with Biomimetic Zones. Tissue Eng Part B Rev. 2009; 15(2):143-57.

[159] Sharma B, Williams CG, Kim TK, Sun D, Malik A, Khan M, Leong K, Elisseeff JH. Designing zonal organization into tissue-engineered cartilage. Tissue Engineering 2007; 13(2): 405-414.

[160] Hwang NS, Varghese S, Lee HJ, Theprungsirikul P, Canver A, Sharma B, Elisseeff J. Response of zonal chondrocytes to extracellular matrix-hydrogels. FEBS Lett. 2007; 581(22):4172–4178.

[161] Melero-Martin, J.M, Al-Rubeai. In N. Ashammakhi, R. L. Reis, E. Chiellini editors. Topics in Tissue Engineering; In Vitro Expansion of Chondrocytes; 2007 (3). http://www.oulu.fi/spareparts/ebook_topics_in_t_e_vol3/abstracts/al-rubeai_chapter_01.pdf

[162] Unterman SA, Gibson M, Lee JH, Crist J, Chansakul T, Yang EC, Elisseeff JH. Hyaluronic Acid-Binding Scaffold for Articular Cartilage Repair. Tissue Eng Part A. 2012; doi:10.1089/ten.tea.2011.0711

[163] Concaro S, Nicklasson E, Ellowsson L, Lindahl A, Brittberg M, Gatenholm P. Effect of cell seeding concentration on the quality of tissue engineered constructs loaded with adult human articular chondrocytes. J Tissue Eng Regen Med. 2008; 2(1):14-21.

[164] Chen FH, Rousche KT, Tuan RS. Technology Insight: adult stem cells in cartilage regeneration and tissue engineering. Nat Clin Pract Rheumatol. 2006; 2(7): 373-82.

[165] Zhang L, Hu J, Athanasiou KA. The Role of Tissue Engineering in Articular Cartilage Repair and Regeneration. Crit Rev Biomed Eng. 2009; 37(1-2): 1–57.

[166] Johnson K, Zhu S, Tremblay MS, Payette JN, Wang J, Bouchez LC, Meeusen S, Althage A, Cho CY, Wu X, Schultz PG. A stem cell-based approach to cartilage repair. Science. 2012; 336 (6082): 717-721.

[167] Chen T, Buckley M, Cohen I, Bonassar L, Awad HA. Insights into interstitial flow, shear stress, and mass transport effects on ECM heterogeneity in bioreactor-cultivated engineered cartilage hydrogels. Biomech Model Mechanobiol. 2012; 11(5):689-702.

[168] McMahon L.A, Barron, V., Prina-Mello, A. In P.J. Prendergast and P.E. McHugh editors. Topics in Bio-Mechanical Engineering – The state-of-the-art in cartilage bioreactors. Trinity Centre for Bioengineering & the National Centre for Biomedical Engineering Science, 2004; 94-146. http://www.tcd.ie/bioengineering/documents/ChapterIV.pdf

[169] Responte DJ, Natoli RM, Athanasiou KA. Identification of potential biophysical and molecular signalling mechanisms underlying hyaluronic acid enhancement of cartilage formation. Soc. Interface, 2012; doi:10.1098/rsif.2012.0399

Permissions

The contributors of this book come from diverse backgrounds, making this book a truly international effort. This book will bring forth new frontiers with its revolutionizing research information and detailed analysis of the nascent developments around the world.

We would like to thank José A. Andrades, for lending his expertise to make the book truly unique. He has played a crucial role in the development of this book. Without his invaluable contribution this book wouldn't have been possible. He has made vital efforts to compile up to date information on the varied aspects of this subject to make this book a valuable addition to the collection of many professionals and students.

This book was conceptualized with the vision of imparting up-to-date information and advanced data in this field. To ensure the same, a matchless editorial board was set up. Every individual on the board went through rigorous rounds of assessment to prove their worth. After which they invested a large part of their time researching and compiling the most relevant data for our readers. Conferences and sessions were held from time to time between the editorial board and the contributing authors to present the data in the most comprehensible form. The editorial team has worked tirelessly to provide valuable and valid information to help people across the globe.

Every chapter published in this book has been scrutinized by our experts. Their significance has been extensively debated. The topics covered herein carry significant findings which will fuel the growth of the discipline. They may even be implemented as practical applications or may be referred to as a beginning point for another development. Chapters in this book were first published by InTech; hereby published with permission under the Creative Commons Attribution License or equivalent.

The editorial board has been involved in producing this book since its inception. They have spent rigorous hours researching and exploring the diverse topics which have resulted in the successful publishing of this book. They have passed on their knowledge of decades through this book. To expedite this challenging task, the publisher supported the team at every step. A small team of assistant editors was also appointed to further simplify the editing procedure and attain best results for the readers.

Our editorial team has been hand-picked from every corner of the world. Their multi-ethnicity adds dynamic inputs to the discussions which result in innovative outcomes. These outcomes are then further discussed with the researchers and contributors who give their valuable feedback and opinion regarding the same. The feedback is then collaborated with the researches and they are edited in a comprehensive manner to aid the understanding of the subject.

Apart from the editorial board, the designing team has also invested a significant amount of their time in understanding the subject and creating the most relevant covers. They scrutinized every image to scout for the most suitable representation of the subject and create an appropriate cover for the book.

The publishing team has been involved in this book since its early stages. They were actively engaged in every process, be it collecting the data, connecting with the contributors or procuring relevant information. The team has been an ardent support to the editorial, designing and production team. Their endless efforts to recruit the best for this project, has resulted in the accomplishment of this book. They are a veteran in the field of academics and their pool of knowledge is as vast as their experience in printing. Their expertise and guidance has proved useful at every step. Their uncompromising quality standards have made this book an exceptional effort. Their encouragement from time to time has been an inspiration for everyone.

The publisher and the editorial board hope that this book will prove to be a valuable piece of knowledge for researchers, students, practitioners and scholars across the globe.

List of Contributors

M. Arnal-Pastor and A. Vallés-Lluch
Center for Biomaterials and Tissue Engineering, Universitat Politècnica de València, Cno, de Vera s/n, Valencia, Spain

J. C. Chachques
Department of Cardiovascular Surgery, Laboratory of Biosurgical Research, Georges Pompidou European Hospital, Paris, France

M. Monleón Pradas
Center for Biomaterials and Tissue Engineering, Universitat Politècnica de València, Cno, de Vera s/n, Valencia, Spain
Networking Research Center on Bioengineering, Biomaterials and Nanomedicine (CIBERBBN), Valencia, Spain

Aleksandar Evangelatov and Roumen Pankov
Department of Cytology, Histology and Embryology, Sofia University "St. Kliment Ohridski", Sofia, Bulgaria

Tran Le Bao Ha, To Minh Quan, Doan Nguyen Vu and Do Minh Si
University of Science, Vietnam National University – Hochiminh city, Vietnam

Dragica Smrke, Matjaž Veselko and Borut Gubina
Department of Surgery, University Medical Center Ljubljana, Ljubljana, Slovenia

Primož Rožman
Blood Transfusion Centre of Slovenia, Ljubljana, Slovenia

Hans- H. Sievers and Norbert W. Guldner
Clinic of Cardiac Surgery, University of Lübeck, Germany

Peter Klapproth
Microstim GmbH, Wismar, Germany

Hangörg Zimmermann
Pfm Titan GmbH Nürnberg, Hangörg Zimmermann, Germany

Qiong Li, Lu Zhang, Guangdong Zhou, Wei Liu and Yilin Cao
Department of Plastic and Reconstructive Surgery, Shanghai the People's Hospital, Shanghai
Jiao Tong University School of Medicine, Shanghai Key Laboratory of Tissue Engineering, Shanghai, P.R. China

Zaira Y. García-Carvajal, David Garciadiego-Cázares, Carmen Parra-Cid and Rocío Aguilar-Gaytán
Tissue Engineering, Cell Therapy and Regenerative Medicine Unit, Instituto Nacional de Rehabilitación, Secretaria de Salud, Mexico city, Mexico

Clemente Ibarra
Tissue Engineering, Cell Therapy and Regenerative Medicine Unit, Instituto Nacional de Rehabilitación, Secretaria de Salud, Mexico city, Mexico
Orthopaedic Surgery and Arthroscopy Servicie, Instituto Nacional de Rehabilitación, Secretaria de Salud, Mexico city, Mexico

Cristina Velasquillo
Biotechnology Laboratory, Centro Nacional de Investigación y Atención al Quemado, Instituto Nacional de Rehabilitación, Secretaria de Salud, Mexico city, Mexico

Javier S. Castro Carmona
Instituto de Ingenieria y Tecnologia, Universidad Autónoma de Ciudad Juárez, Juarez City, Chihuahua, Mexico

Printed in the USA
CPSIA information can be obtained
at www.ICGtesting.com
JSHW011357221024
72173JS00003B/319

9 781632 412447